D0983360

Sleep Disorders:

Insomnia and Narcolepsy

by

HENRY KELLERMAN, Ph.D.

Postgraduate Center for Mental Health
New York, N.Y.

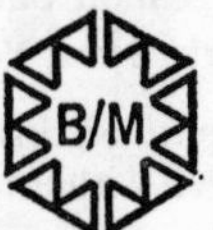

BRUNNER/MAZEL, *Publishers* • New York

Library of Congress Cataloging in Publication Data

Kellerman, Henry.
Sleep disorders.
Bibliography: p.
Includes index.

1. Insomnia. 2. Narcolepsy. I. Title.
[DNLM: 1. Insomnia. 2. Narcolepsy. WM 188 L29s]
RC548.K44 616.8'49 80-28517
ISBN 0-87630-264-9

Copyright © 1981 by HENRY KELLERMAN

Published by
BRUNNER/MAZEL, INC.
19 Union Square
New York, New York 10003

All rights reserved. No part of this book may be reproduced by any process whatsoever without the written permission of the copyright owner.

MANUFACTURED IN THE UNITED STATES OF AMERICA

To

LINDA, MAX, SAM, HARRY, JACK

Preface

In the United States of America alone, estimates of persons with sleep problems range from a low of 10 million to a high of 50 million. It has only been in the past decade that scientists have produced a sea of facts and information on the nature of sleep. Yet this information is not widely disseminated or readily available to the professional person. It is also not usually the kind of information that can offer physicians and psychotherapists comprehensive and cogent guidance in helping problem sleepers to sleep better. The net effect of such fragmentation is that professional practitioners frequently find themselves operating with only a marginal grasp of sleep disorders generally, and insomnia and narcolepsy specifically.

In the past 23 years I have had the opportunity to work with patients who have suffered from insomnia—the inability to sleep—and from narcolepsy—the compelling need to sleep. The overriding complaint made by people who suffer with these problems is the difficulty they have faced over many years in acquiring any relevant treatment regimen. Such sleep sufferers also lament the virtual absence of any significant reading material that could have shed some light on their particular sleep problems—a complaint not unlike that made by physicians and psychotherapists.

Recently, several national and local media events targeted for both professional and lay audiences have focused on the problems of insomnia and narcolepsy. One was a Public Broadcasting System televised phonathon concerning sleep problems. The audience response was astounding, indicating that: 1) both physicians and psychotherapists, as well as the general public, are profoundly underinformed about the many varieties of sleep problems; and 2) these problems afflict many more people, perhaps millions more, than had been assumed.

Another media event was a three-day 15-hour radio program, broadcast by WKCR-FM (New York) on the problems of narcolepsy. This program included interviews with several experts on narcolepsy, an interview with a narcoleptic person, and a call-in hot line that enabled listeners to participate. A staggering statistic to emerge from this broadcast was that it usually takes from four to six consultations with different physicians over a period of 10 to 15 years before the accurate diagnosis of a narcoleptic condition is made. This has meant that narcoleptic persons were often erroneously treated for conditions variously labeled hypoglycemia, schizophrenia, depression, hypothyroidism, "housewife syndrome," and hysterical psychosis; in addition, they were often called lazy, unmotivated, non-productive and ineffectual. There are even cases where narcoleptic persons were hospitalized for schizophrenia and released only after the misdiagnosis became apparent. The current estimates of the number of narcoleptics range from one-quarter of a million to a million. However, there may be three to five million narcoleptics in this country alone who show only some of the narcoleptic symptoms. It is further estimated that in the United States there are more narcoleptic persons than those, for example, with either muscular dystrophy or Parkinson's disease.

In 1979, the journal *Psychiatric Annals* devoted two full issues to the problem of sleep, with a special focus on insomnia, narcolepsy, sleep apnea and the general associated problem of depression. This unprecedented attention to the problem of sleep provides a clear signal of the acute concern felt by the medical and psychological helping professions regarding the epidemic nature of this problem. In fact, a crash program has begun to educate practitioners in the treatment of such problems.

> "To enhance physicians' knowledge of the prevalent problem of sleep disorders, a 50-minute videotape program designed as a learning and self assessment experience in evaluating and treating these disorders was coproduced with the Network for Continuing Medical Education. This program has been presented nationally to about 25 thousand medical professionals and allied health professionals and over 800 medical institutions in all 50 states. The large size of the audience, its wide distribution, and the representation of different types of physicians and allied health professionals indicate that there is an active interest in this type of program as well as the need for clinically relevant education in sleep disorders" (Kales, Kales, Bixter & Soldatos, 1979).

In another study (Bixler, Kales, Scharf, et al., 1976), it is reported that physicians state that no less than one-quarter of all their patients complain of sleep problems. Ware (1979) even claims that there are up to 75 million people in the United States who complain of sleep difficulties.

In response to this acute need for education and research on sleep problems, many sleep study research centers have sprung up throughout the country in the past five to ten years and have joined in the formation of the Association of Sleep Disorder Centers. In addition, the film *Keep Us Awake* is also being widely shown to lay as well as professional audiences.

For all these reasons, I have written this book in the hope that it will fill the need for a comprehensive reference book on insomnia and narcolepsy for the physician, the professional mental health worker, as well as students in medical and graduate schools. It is a psychodynamically oriented work and relates personality factors to biological aspects of sleep disorders.

I have treated the subject matter of insomnia, narcolepsy and other sleep problems under three general headings: etiology, diagnosis, and treatment. Under *etiology,* sleep problems are considered with respect to: a review of theories of causation; a presentation of the psychophysiology of sleep and its role in the appearance of specific sleep problems; theories of psychological problems associated with sleep disorders; and both physiological and biological involvement in the onset of such problems. Within the framework of *diagnosis,* sleep problems are reviewed with respect to: an analysis of symptoms and syndromes of specific sleep disorders; a comparison of psychological diagnoses associated with sleep disorders with that of other diagnostic syndromes; and a presentation of ways to identify sleep problems with the events that have triggered them. In terms of *treatment,* specific sleep disorders are examined with respect to: psychological testing and corresponding psychotherapy intervention; drug treatment and its short- and long-term effects, along with an analysis of side effects.

Clinical illustrations and case studies are offered throughout to further amplify the issues considered under all three headings: etiology, diagnosis, and treatment. Finally, the many types of sleep problems are unified by a general theory of the historical underpinnings of these problems.

My intention has been to suggest that sleep problems may be modified and controlled. I have tried to show how this might be done. The assumption of this book is that if one understands the conditions that have generated such problems and is knowledgeable about the specific biological and psychological nature of particular sleep disorders, then a first important step can be taken to control them. To this end, the practitioner can read this book: 1) to develop a psychological orientation and help locate the cause of a patient's sleep difficulties; 2) to utilize such insights to begin to control specific problems of sleep; and 3) to utilize information about the physiology of sleep to better administer treatment aids, whether chemical or psychological.

The book is divided into four parts. Part I presents an introduction to two main issues involved in the development of disordered sleep—an analysis of those individual personality features that contribute to sleep problems and those reciprocal interpersonal phenomena inherent in the onset of these disorders. These variables are central in the genesis of both narcolepsy and insomnia.

Part II presents the entire narcoleptic condition with respect to psychological as well as physiological phenomena. This topic is discussed first because it provides a framework for more readily understanding the scope of the field of sleep research as it relates to sleep aberration, dream disruption, and the physiology of the sleep cycle.

The more familiar sleep problem of insomnia is presented in Part III. Here, the entire variety of insomnias are analyzed within the context of normal versus abnormal physiological sleep. Special topics of interest related to insomnia are also considered, including issues concerned with chronobiological or "inner clock" phenomena, an analysis of the sleep cycle, and an introduction to sleep apnea as a special kind of sleep problem.

The final section of the volume, Part IV, offers a synthesis of the theoretical aspects of insomnia and narcolepsy that have been discussed throughout the book. In addition, I have presented the case of a sleep-disordered family treated in a family setting.

Throughout the book the discussion of narcolepsy and insomnia will also focus on problems or elements of sleep disorders associated with the four major sleep disorder categories listed in the *Diagnostic Classification of Sleep and Arousal Disorders* (1979). These are: Disorders of Initiating and Maintaining Sleep, Disorders of Excessive Somnolence, Disorders of the Sleep-Wake Schedule, and, Dysfunctions Associated with Sleep, Sleep Stages or Partial Arousals.

Acknowledgments

Several of my colleagues, representing a wide clinical and scientific range of interdisciplinary specialties, have critically reviewed various aspects of this book. Their individual expertise in theory, research, and treatment has been exceedingly helpful in shaping the final form of the manuscript.

In this regard I would like to thank: Dr. Anthony Burry, who reviewed sections of the manuscript relating to clinical diagnoses and the reporting of psychological test results; Dr. Abraham I. Cohen, who reviewed the sections on depression and insomnia; Dr. Milton Klein, who reviewed material on object-relations theory; Dr. Robert Lampert, who evaluated the manuscript with respect to theoretical aspects of etiology in the onset of sleep disorders; Dr. Alvaro Rozo-Sanmiguel, who checked the reporting and analyses of psychopharmacological aspects of treatment; and, Dr. Robert Plutchik, who made useful comments concerning the material on neurophysiology and on the experimental studies reported.

The typing of the manuscript was accomplished with skill and care and I would like to thank Ms. Tracy Bailey, Ms. Hannah Otten, and Ms. Joan Sullivan for their help in that regard. As always, Ms. Lee Mackler, Chief Librarian and Ms. Carol Strauss, Assistant Librarian of the Postgraduate Center for Mental Health were extremely helpful in the location of important materials and citations.

Finally, to all of the patients with sleep problems that I have treated over the years goes my sincere appreciation for allowing me to simultaneously help and learn.

Contents

Part I

EVOLUTIONARY AND PSYCHOLOGICAL SIGNIFICANCE OF SLEEP

Chapter 1

The Primary Cause of Sleep Problems

THE BASIC MEANING OF SLEEP

During the course of history, the nature of relationships developed within the framework of group living. The success of group life was reflected in the increased survival potential of each member of the group. As group living became more and more complex, attachments and relationships created an ever increasing community of interest among people, thereby reinforcing reciprocal bondings. This community of interest also implied that people could sleep with ever increasing security (Dement, 1972). The partial equation that can be applied to this bonding phenomenon is that good sleep and existing bonds between people go together. Thus, group living allowed sleeping to be more pleasurable and not subject to any great threat. Dement (1972) points out that

> "Night was once man's enemy. . . . Perhaps family life itself originated from the need to sleep and to cluster for protection while in this state. . . . Because sleep occurs during the dark hours when man is least able to cope with his environment and because man asleep is not alert to the dangers of the outer world, sleep is a state of vulnerability. . . . It is necessary to seek a place of refuge in which to sleep. A troop of baboons has its

tree, the wolf has its den, primitive man had his cave or his hut, and we have our bedrooms."

Dement further shows the connection between sleep and relationships by displaying a series of Picasso prints entitled *The Sleeper Watched*. This series consists of many different paintings in which one person of a pair sleeps while the other watches. This sense that relationships and sleep developed around the need for protection is also pointed out by Gutheil (1951) who traces the derivation of the word sleep from the German *wachen—to be awake*. However, *wache* means *guard*. Thus, the consequences of sleeping alone included the possibility that one could be susceptible to attack.

In terms of such possible attack, sleep also contains mechanisms that have presumably developed for protective purposes. For example, the entire sleep cycle is one in which a person gradually falls deeper and deeper into sleep and then gradually emerges from deep sleep into light sleep (Dement and Mitler, 1973; Hartmann, 1970; Kleitman, 1963; and, Williams, Karacan and Hirsch, 1974). This oscillation occurs throughout the night. It suggests that even while asleep a person can have greater periodic access to the external world whenever the sleep cycle generates the shallow phase of sleep. This shallow phase of the sleep cycle, when a person can be awakened by the slightest noise, also developed as an adaptive protective mechanism. The sense of needing to be guarded during sleep may also correspond to the development of paranoid suspiciousness—that is, a guarded attitude characteristic of some withdrawn and perhaps critical people with whom the term paranoid is associated.

In certain respects, then, the shallow phase of the sleep cycle, when people can be awakened by the slightest disturbance, can be attributed to the need for protection as this need was etched into the evolution of the entire sleep cycle. Just as good sleep and bonding between people form a partial equation, so too does poor sleep and separation from bonding complete the equation. The basic idea expressed throughout this book is that *existing relationships and good sleep go together and broken relationships and poor sleep go together.*

Gutheil further proposes that insomnia is related to the individual's connection to others, while hypersomnia—the abnormal desire to sleep—is similarly related to dissatisfaction in one's life, especially with respect to an escape from emptiness or loneliness. Freud also referred to sleep being impeded by powerful emotions or the "unfinished business" of emotions; he saw wish fulfillment as a reflection of the unfinished business of interpersonal relationships. Thus, through historical development, the mechanisms and nature of sleep became inextricably associated with attachment to other people.

THE SYMBOLIC TRAPPINGS OF SLEEP

There are many variations of this sleep-related theme of togetherness versus separation. For example, in various cultures it is a widespread practice for newborns to be snugly wrapped after birth. This procedure will immediately comfort the newborn infant. The experience of being swaddled is obviously akin to being hugged or touched. Apparently, through evolution, a sense of security has been built into skin-to-skin, or touch-to-touch, contact. This creature contact need has been aptly captured in several little poems reported by Harlow (1958)* which make the point convincingly.

The Rhinoceros

The rhino's skin is thick and tough. And yet
this skin is soft enough that baby rhinos
always sense, A love enormous and intense.

The Hippopotamus

This is the skin some babies feel
Replete with hippo love appeal
Each contact, cuddle, push and shove
Elicits tons of baby love.

The Elephant

Though mother may be short on arms,
Her skin is full of warmth and charms,
And mother's touch on baby's skin
Endears the heart that beats within.

* Copyright 1958 by the American Psychological Association. Reprinted by permission.

The Crocodile

Here is the skin they love to touch.
It isn't soft and there isn't much,
But its contact comfort will beguile
Love from the infant crocodile.

In all of these vignettes, the importance of loving contact with a significant other person is quite simply portrayed. The need for this kind of contact has also been absorbed into the rituals and trappings of sleep. Individuals bid each other good night upon going to sleep; if alone and watching television, an individual may find comfort, at the end of the program day, by an announcer's wish for a good, peaceful or happy night. Furthermore, comforting feelings arise from being tucked in or from the weight of covers and the feel of soft pillows. It may be suggested that the use of pillows in the first place, or the use of some other head rest, is a symbolic expression of sleeping especially close to someone. The pillow represents another person, in addition to its practical use as a postural and respiratory aid.

> A patient suffering from insomnia remarked that she could occasionally overcome her inability to fall asleep if she tucked herself in from head to toe and used an abundance of comforters and pillows. Her tension would then subside and she would gradually drift off to sleep. She was a single, middle-aged woman.

One way to understand this phenomenon is to suggest that when this woman slept with comforters and pillows and was all tucked in, it consoled her in some vaguely conscious manner and anesthetized her sense of utter isolation and despair. When she eliminated all arid reminders, she no longer was confronted by symbols of separation. In the absence of these *separation-reminders* she could gradually fall asleep. This is a typical experience reported by people who feel alone and isolated and seem to need an abundance of pillows and comforters. Such examples suggest that sleep problems can be set off by some inadequacy of relationships, especially in people who are quite troubled by aspects of dependency.

In the evolution of sleep mechanisms, therefore, sleeping with, near, or next to someone else became associated with attachment and relationship to another specific person. Bonding or pairing was the beginning of the relationship phenomenon, although its roots must have existed in parent-child interactions. An example of this parent-child bonding is given by Bergman (1971) in the study of the treatment of a symbiotic-psychotic child.

> "Rachel's mother suffered from a sleep disturbance which had begun when she was forced to give up her studies and to work at an uninteresting job in order to support herself and her mother. She then began to sleep late, sometimes around the clock, or else she would be completely unable to sleep and her nights would turn into nightmares of anxiety. In order to avoid the pain, she would simply not go to bed. However, her sleep disturbance would vanish completely when she had to care for someone else —for example her dying mother or her helpless infant."

As complexity in relationships developed, so too did the symbiotic or psychological meaning of sleep. A vivid commentary on this proposition is offered by Kupfermann (1971), also in a study on the treatment of a psychotic child.

> "Eric suffered sleep disturbances. . . . He told me that closing his eyes was like saying goodbye . . . falling asleep . . . is an experience of separation."

Finally, in an early, classic study, Kleitman (1939) points out that both animals and people can be induced to fall asleep in response to holding, rocking or cradling, an oblique reference, indeed, to the close correspondence of the nature of sleep with the nature of one's relationships.

It is the thesis of this book, therefore, that although sleep is physiologically determined, it also has developed with psychological meaning or with a symbolic component. This component refers essentially to the idea that one's sleep pattern is directly affected by the state of one's relationships. The idea of the correspondence between sleep and relationships will be developed in the following sections. The basic link between sleep problems and relationships is that if sleep is disturbed, then one's primary relationship may be disturbed; if sleep is undisturbed, then one's primary relationship is likely to be undisturbed.

NORMAL AND PROBLEMATIC RELATIONSHIPS

It should be noted that sometimes one's relationship with another person can be quite troublesome. Nevertheless, even a troublesome or chaotic relationship, if it has lasted many years, is composed of two people, each of whom plays some part in retaining it. Often, people who have the most problematic relationships resist most in changing them. It is important to remember that even an unhealthy relationship may still be one in which both persons sleep quite well. Were these individuals to be separated, however, then one or both could quite likely, and even immediately, develop sleep problems.

The absence of sleep problems, then, implies that one's primary relationship remains intact, whether or not this relationship is healthy or free from severely debilitating problems. *The onset of sleep problems implies that a drastic change has occurred in one's primary relationship.*

An understanding of how sleep corresponds to the nature of one's significant relationship may be gained by examining the sleep of children. Children under the age of 13 are infrequently diagnosed as insomniacs although the incidence in children, of poor sleeping, may be underestimated (Anders and Guilleminault, 1976). Occasional fitful sleeping, difficulties in standardizing sleeping procedures at night, and fear of the dark do not by any means represent problems or profound aspects of sleep disorders. These are all experiences reported by young children, but they do not constitute actual insomnia. This raises the question of why children do not have sleep problems (such as insomnia or hyposomnia) in the same proportions as adults.

There is no definite answer to this question. Physiologically, the sleep-dream cycle of children is relatively stable although children's sleep is deeper and longer than the sleep of adults. There are, however, psychological speculations about the presumed lower incidence of insomnia during childhood. One such speculation would propose that even in tense children there is an absence of profound anxiety with respect to haphazard sleeplessness because the basic relationships of children—meaning their relationships with parents—are more or less intact. The fact that parents instruct and care for the child, who, by definition, is dependent on them, is sufficient to create the circumstances for adequate sleep. As long as the basic dependency patern is maintained, then children as well as adults will tend to sleep well and will not be overly worried about poor sleeping.

> One vivid example of the correspondence between sleeping and the nature of intact relationships was offered by a male patient who was in his mid-forties. He had five children and was deeply in love with his wife. His attachment to his family happened also to be congruent with his tendency to need to rely on other adults around him. He was dependent on his wife's superior judgment in the decision-making process of the family. He sought psychotherapy consultation because his wife could not understand why he would become tense whenever the entire family happened to simultaneously retire for the evening. The patient responded:
>
> "I think I get nervous when we all go to sleep at the same time. It gets too quiet. I can feel my heart start to pound and my mind starts to race. I feel very uncomfortable and have to sit up. On the other hand, when everyone else goes to sleep and I happen to be doing something at the time, I feel better. Then I get the good feeling that everyone is in bed and all is safe and sound. I feel relieved and can go to sleep later on."

Somehow, this man would feel calm knowing his wife was asleep. Psychodynamically, he actually needed to see her sleeping in order to experience the satisfaction of his dependency feelings—perhaps another example of the Picasso theme of the sleeper watched. When they all went to sleep at the same time, he experienced separation. On the other hand, having the opportunity to watch his wife sleep reassured him of her presence.

WHAT IS A PRIMARY RELATIONSHIP?

Since it is being proposed that disturbed sleep is caused by an upset or separation in one's primary relationship, it is necessary to explain what a primary relationship is. A primary relationship is defined as one's closest emotional connection to another person. This may mean a spouse, parent, sibling, friend, boyfriend, girlfriend or child. It may also mean an employer, teacher, or student. In some cases it may even mean a relationship not to another person but to one's job.

Psychoanalysis teaches that each of these possible connections may have roots in earlier relations. For example, one's relationship to a spouse may resemble, in certain important ways, similar early family relationships with one or both parents. Psychoanalysis calls this transference. It means that an individual may tend automatically to react to someone who is close to him in the present in the same manner that he behaved toward a parent when he was a child. For example, a person who was an obedient child—and whose mother was a controlling person requiring the child to do everything exactly her way—may respond obediently in the present to anyone who also seems domineering or controlling. Thus, there is a memory, as it were, of past important relationships that has some influence in affecting present relationships.

An individual's primary relationship may, by implication, threaten the memory of that person's early family relationships. Such a disturbance of primary connections will likely produce a sleep disturbance. For example, if through some significant experience a person were to become defiant instead of typically obedient in responding to the individual with whom one had a primary relationship, then the balance of this current interaction would become upset. This kind of disturbance of the current relationship suggests to each partner that the old way may be jeopardized—it may no longer be possible. Changes such as these sometimes disrupt relationships and produce separations or *separation anxiety*. When that happens, sleep problems are likely to occur.

In terms of the above discussion, an individual's primary relationship may be identified as the one shared with another person most of the time. If one lives with the original family, it is likely to be a parent —usually one's mother. If married, it is likely to be one's spouse. Even when a person is living alone, his or her emotional tie to another, either in the present or in the past, would constitute a closest or primary relationship, and any significant change in the present or historical connection to this person can cause sleep problems.

THE DIFFERENT KINDS OF SEPARATIONS

There are all sorts of separations. Most are real, involving some current person. Others may relate to a person in the past from whom one may begin to feel estranged. The important point about separations is that they come in many different shapes and styles. There are all kinds of separations. The most obvious is marital separation and divorce. Other kinds include death of a loved one, moving away from home, and losing one's job. Each of these can cause a person to feel as though a dreadful event—equivalent to a death—has occurred. Fodor (1949) illustrates this point by citing the case of a 46-year-old man who suffered with severe insomnia starting after his mother died, and, Peretz (1970) in a paper on reaction to loss also indicates that sleep problems typically occur as a response to loss and grief.

Separations always contain a symbolic element of death and loss. Even in a separation that one of the partners welcomes, sleep problems may still occur simply because that partner has not been accustomed to living alone. The presence of a sleeping partner is generally reassuring even though problems may exist in one's relationship to that person. Good sleeping means being *with* someone. Leaving or being left by someone may trigger poor sleeping or too much sleeping.

Separation from one's family may cause sleep problems. Some authors have pointed out that the onset of narcolepsy occurred when the patient moved away from the parents' home. Furthermore, if a son or daughter who is highly dependent on a parent vehemently argues with that parent to the point of perceiving a rupture in their relationship, then sudden and even severe insomnia may appear in both the dependent child and the parent. The emotions of fear and anger are frequently observed in persons suffering from insomnia of this sort. The fear of solitude as well as anger directed toward the separated person are emotions that occur simultaneously with such problems of separation and insomnia.

The loss of a job can also cause sleep problems. This kind of event can create extreme financial anxieties that also raise the possibility of creating separations and fragmentations in one's life. The loss of a job also leads to insomnia because the basic transference to the job, or the basic attitude toward it, contains ingredients that resemble those of early family relationships. The feelings of loss or separation from such relationships can generate intense anxieties contributing to one's general distress with respect to the lost job.

Insomnia, as a clinical syndrome, is different from simple temporary disturbance of sleep. Insomnia should be a two- or three-month uninterrupted symptom before it can be considered entrenched. A restless night or two does not constitute insomnia. The level of a person's emotional maturity will determine how well any separation storm can be weathered. For the most part, emotional maturity develops from the experiences of early family relationships. The less difficult or less problematic these experiences, the better adjustment one can make to separation later on. The more difficult or more problematic these early experiences were, the poorer may be the adjustment to separation, and the more likely it may be for sleep problems to emerge.

Anyone's level of emotional maturity depends in large measure on the extent to which that person learned to be independent during formative years (Winnicott, 1953, 1958). Emotional maturity, however, does not depend solely on whether someone was loved. To be emotionally mature and able to cope with separation implies that the caring one experienced while growing up was not of a smothering sort. Overprotective love breeds petulance and reinforces dependency needs; it generates a poor ability to cope with separation in later life. In such cases, severe and enduring sleep problems may develop with respect to a wide variety of life's conditions—especially with regard to separation experiences. The main point is that the more independent a person was during formative years, the better chance that person has to cope with separations of all sorts in the present. Yet, personality structure can be very resilient and even if early life experiences were problematic, a great deal can be done in the present to combat and ultimately defeat any insomnia condition.

THE DEPENDENT TYPE: A POTENTIAL PROBLEM SLEEPER

The one type of person who is highly susceptible to sleep problems is the *dependent* type—the person who has always been highly reliant on parents or parental figures for guidance and decision making. It is primarily this kind of person who finds it difficult to manage the anxieties caused by separation experiences. Identifying the extent to which a person is dependent is not always easy. Sometimes someone who seems to be the independent partner in a relationship is really the one who depends on the other partner's presence for security. Most often, however, a dependent partner in a relationship can be identified as the one who serves the other. The following case illustrates how early historical experiences generated and reinforced intense dependency needs.

> A highly intelligent man of 38 initially came to therapy because he could not sleep. It quickly became evident that his sleep problem was related to a recent separation from his girlfriend, after which he suddenly developed insomnia. It was also soon revealed that as a child he was almost totally dependent upon his mother. She was a gregarious and non-introspective woman who would help him with his problems by saying things like, "Don't worry, if you just do your homework then people will like you," or, "Things work out for the best," or, "Leave it to me."
>
> This man grew up on a sense of mother-superstition. An independent impulse never seemed to awaken in him and he would always rely on some encouraging wishful thought from his mother to alleviate his anxieties. His tension would subside after such magical stroking, but things hardly ever worked out for him.
>
> Ten years before his current sleep problem occurred, at the age of 28, he moved away from home and developed his first experience of insomnia. This insomnia lasted about five years.

> It was a condition that subsided when he developed a relationship with a woman who was several years older than he. After that, each time his relationships with women would end, he would experience a problem in sleeping. This current episode was just another, in a long line of problems with insomnia that were related to separations from women on whom he was highly dependent, as he had been on his mother.

This case underscores the prevalence of dependency symptoms typically seen in severe problem sleepers. In such cases, the effects of separation anxiety are so great that such persons will stop sleeping or they will oversleep, in some cases up to 18 hours a day. Those who oversleep can eventually also become insomniacs. Their initial oversleeping is generally an unsuccessful attempt, as Gutheil (1951) indicates, to escape ravages of separation or impending separation experiences.

Any type of separation can cause insomnia in persons who are intensely dependent. A woman who sleeps well whenever her lover is present but experiences severe insomnia when he is absent is an example frequently reported. There are also many cases reported of married men maintaining separate apartments for single women who, in turn, spend their time literally waiting for these men to appear. These women are generally highly dependent and frequently need tranquilizing or special sleep medication to help control their insomnia. Separation in marriage is, of course, fertile ground for the appearance of insomnia. A third type of insomnia-related problem concerns individuals who are chronologically mature adults still living at home with their original families. These persons may develop insomnia if there is a breach in their inordinate dependency relationship with parents.

Another form of insomnia is observed in individuals who have never really satisfied their deep dependency needs to be cared for and supervised, and continue to yearn for such gratification. Generally, they will be very angry with those family members who originally frustrated them, but will continue to seek them out for the same purpose that they could not fulfill in the past. Even when they do try to establish a mature relationship, the historical expectation is that primary love and dependency needs will never be met.

> Despite repeated expressions of love and loyalty from his girlfriend, a male patient in his late 30's could not believe that these expressions were real. He would always find something to complain about and to feel deprived about. His only reality was the recollection of his childhood experience in which he would lie awake at night calling in vain for his mother. His need was never met. He acted in the present with feelings that had been determined in the past and no amount of real love could affect him. He could not believe that he would ever be loved. He was an inveterate insomniac who virtually lived on tranquilizing and sleep medications.

Apparently this man could not permit anyone to reach him for fear of becoming vulnerable to their whims and this accounted for his critical stance. He would not allow anyone to be with him and therefore no one could leave him.

COMPONENTS OF DEPENDENCY

The effects of separation reveal important components of dependency problems. Following are examples of six significant characteristics in the personalities of highly dependent individuals who are potential problem sleepers.

First, dependent persons generally react strongly to separation or threats of separation and have low tolerance for frustration. For example, those who are more susceptible to insomnia frequently become angry when frustrated. They can become vindictive or spiteful. In so doing, they may, in effect, stubbornly refuse to work out whatever the problem is and their overabundance of rage can cause psychosomatic symptoms such as migraine headaches. On the other hand, dependent persons who become resigned in the face of frustration or become depressed, may simply withdraw into sleep.

Second, dependent persons tend to rely on magical solutions for their problems—they may wish for someone to suddenly appear and solve their problems for them, or they may believe that somehow things will work out.

> One young woman who was frustrated in her never ending quest for a husband declared that she would contemplate suicide if somehow she did not get *a sign* that she would meet a man.

Third, dependent persons have identified with the style of the parent on whom they are dependent, so that they too behave in this fatefully optimistic and usually self-defeating way.

Fourth, such persons, whether or not they are accomplished, do not trust their achievements. They tend to minimize them and they usually attribute all accomplishments to some unexpected luck.

> One woman claimed that her success as a tennis player was directly related to her vomiting before a match. She would intentionally throw up before each match in order to feel confident of winning. This sort of magical and obsessive-compulsive behavior prevented her from appreciating any of her accomplishments and revealed her basic dependent attitude.

Fifth, severely dependent persons are frequently *symbiotic* and not well enough *differentiated*. What this means is not only that such persons find themselves in a dependent-reliant relationship with a parent, but that the parent is similarly locked into the same dependent-reliant pattern. The net effect of this two way neurosis is that the dependent one who is a potential problem sleeper does not ever really have a chance to know where the parent ends and he or she begins. Such individuals cannot then differentiate themselves from their parents. Dependent potential problem sleepers, thus, do not visualize themselves as distinctly different from their parents, and this greater sense of undifferentiated self is the bedrock of the dependency problem.

Sixth, severely dependent persons are frequently socially fearful. They are afraid of confrontations and will construct the most convoluted tales in order to avoid direct encounters with other people. Asking someone the simplest direct question can be embarrassing and extremely difficult for such individuals.

> One 25-year-old man walked over 100 city blocks to his destination because he was too embarrassed to ask a train conductor for directions. Although his capacity to walk that distance also suggests determination, it nevertheless gains its initial momentum from dependency feelings and immature social development.

Individuals with the above characteristics of dependency are more vulnerable to sleep problems. Such persons may develop insomnia problems in response to separations while others may develop withdrawal sleep symptoms and may even show bona-fide narcoleptic problems, also as a result of such separation experiences. Dependent persons with sleep problems will frequently also develop depressive symptoms as well as sexual problems during times of separations. These will be considered later in Chapter 12 in the discussion of depression and sleep.

Persons who are severely dependent and singularly unable to cope with separations are also always searching for conditions that can offer them the emotional security they so desperately crave. Attainment of such security feelings is important because they can resemble original family conditions that offered a great sense of security. During any separation from such a relationship in the present, the severly dependent separated partner is truly alone, and sleep is the arena in which the effect of this problem emerges.

When the needed dependency relationship is intact, a person may not experience any problem of sleep whatsoever. An intact, intense dependency relationship is enough to prevent any sleep problem from occurring even when temporary separations, such as vacations, occur. An undisturbed historical relationship in which dependency needs were successfully met is also one that can continue to nourish good sleep. Any disturbance of such a memory, however, can cause sleep problems.

> A single woman who had just turned 40 developed symptoms in which she could not swallow her food and could not sleep at night. After several therapy sessions, she described a recent visit with an old family friend who confessed to her that she had conducted a 20-year affair with the patient's father. This patient, who revered her father on whom she had been extremely de-

> pendent, maintained an idealized image of him. Even though he had died more than five years earlier, her dependence on her father was carried on in her fantasy and the mere memory of their father-favorite daughter relationship was enough to sustain this woman through all adversity. She had never before experienced a sleep problem. However, now that her father's perfect image was sullied, the unwanted revelation about his indiscretion created a symbolic break in their relationship—a separation between them—and this woman instantly developed several psychiatric symptoms as well as a severe condition of insomnia.

This clinical illustration shows that one's closest relationship may not even be living in the same house, or, for that matter, may not even be alive at all; yet the psychological conditions that produce sleep problems can be triggered by fantasy and memory.

WILL SEPARATION ANXIETY PRODUCE SLEEP PROBLEMS IN ALL KINDS OF PEOPLE?

The question becomes, are severely dependent people the only ones to develop sleep problems as an effect of separation anxiety? The answer to this question is that sleep, in terms of its emotional sense and its symbolic meaning, is related to the nature of one's important relationships. Any disturbance of such important relationships, therefore, will probably generate some sleep problem. This cause and effect between relationship disturbances and sleep disorders is normal. In severely dependent people, the sleep problem may appear more quickly, last longer and generally cause greater anxiety. In more independent people—those who are more maturely adjusted and more relaxed about handling of life's challenges—disturbance in an important relationship will also cause sleep problems, but these will probably not appear as quickly, will not last as long, and will not produce the intense anxiety seen in more dependent types.

The attachment of dependent types on their partners is of a different sort than the attachments more mature people have. Wretmark (1959) indicates, for example, that the more immature person experiences greater difficulty in managing loss. When a separation occurs in the significant relationship of a severely dependent person, it may feel as though one has been set adrift on a stormy sea. It must be remembered that dependent persons rely on their significant relationships for total emotional security and perceive such relationships to be necessary for life itself.

The more dependent the person, the more incomplete is personality formation. For the dependent person to feel complete, attachments must be secure. The achievement of such dependency will assure relatively sound sleep. When such successful achievement of dependency is interfered with, as during times of serious separations, then sleep problems will surely develop.

The actual onset, development and treatment of both insomnia and narcolepsy proper will be described in the following chapters.

Part II

NARCOLEPSY

Chapter 2

Narcolepsy: The Sleep Attack Problem

WHAT IS NARCOLEPSY?

Narcolepsy was first diagnosed in the latter half of the 19th century by Gélineau (1880) although it has been traced to Greco-Roman medicine (Jelliffe, 1930). It was originally defined as an inexorable desire to sleep that may occur anytime and anyplace. A person with narcolepsy may be sitting at a desk, on a couch watching T.V., driving a car, or sometimes even holding a conversation; yet a compelling and irresistible urge to sleep can overpower that person's will to stay awake.

What typically occurs is that an overwhelming need to sleep suddenly emerges. The narcoleptic sleep instantly takes over. One can see the narcoleptic's eyes roll up into his/her head even before this person's lids are fully closed. The eyes then slowly close while sleep hypnotically triumphs.

The narcoleptic sleep is frequently misdiagnosed as neurasthenia, lethargy, general fatigue, and even depression. However, narcolepsy proper is not simply too much sleep as in the case of people tending to withdraw through extra sleep. Narcolepsy is most frequently a kind of sleep that is short. Sometimes the sleep of a narcoleptic may last 60 seconds and sometimes it could last 10 minutes. However, some authors report narcoleptic attacks that have lasted for one hour or longer (Guilleminault, 1976; Rechtschaffen, Wolpert and Dement, 1963; Roberts, 1970). Other case studies are reported by Pond (1952) and the syndrome is described in Dement, Rechtschaffen, and Gulevich (1966); and, Ganado (1958). Narcolepsy is now clearly recognized as a pathophysiological central nervous system condition (Diagnostic Classification of Sleep and Arousal Disorders, 1979).

As the narcoleptic uncontrolled sleep attack occurs, it becomes immediately apparent to anyone observing it. The attack resembles a sleep drunkenness. A very good description of this sleep drunkenness is offered by Kleitman (1963).

> ". . . eyes become heavy and dull, pupils smaller—head inclines. He may attempt to raise his head, gazing rather stupidly at the observer meanwhile, but after a few vain efforts his eyes close and he has every appearance of being soundly asleep."

The narcoleptic firmly believes that any sleep attack can be hidden or disguised so that others would not notice it. This belief is self-delusional. The narcoleptic can never really hide a sleep attack. Almost everyone who is in some way even slightly associated with this person will notice the sleep drunkenness during the onset of an attack. The fallacy of the narcoleptic's belief in the potential success of preventing the sleep attack permits all others to witness the attack while the narcoleptic is hopelessly trying to fight it.

The narcoleptic's uncontrolled sleep episode is not the only true symptom of this disorder. There are three other major symptoms and a fifth associated one that together comprise the picture of the classic narcoleptic. The four basic symptoms are called the *narcoleptic tetrad* (Yoss and Daly, 1957; Zarcone, 1973). In the Diagnostic Classification of Sleep and Arousal Disorders (1979) narcolepsy is listed as a Disorder Of Excessive Somnolence (DOES).

Not all narcoleptics experience each of the major four symptoms, but many do. The narcoleptic tetrad includes: (1) the narcoleptic uncontrolled *sleep attack* described above; (2) an attack of *cataplexy* —episodes of complete muscular weakness in which the narcoleptic's voluntary muscular control becomes inhibited and the person may collapse like a bodyless heap of clothing falling to the floor; (3) an attack of *sleep paralysis* during which the narcoleptic person, when about to fall asleep or awaken, becomes paralyzed and cannot move, and (4) a sleep paralysis, during which the person may experience *hypnagogic hallucinations*. This means that during the sleep paralysis a dream-like state will occur in which the dream scenario becomes so vivid and seems so terribly real that when this person finally awakens,

TABLE 2.1

The Narcoleptic Tetrad and Syndrome

Symptom	*Description*
Narcoleptic Sleep Attack	Sleep drunkenness and uncontrolled excessive daytime sleepiness (E.D.S.) occurs. Actual sleeping occurs throughout the day with sleep-onset REM period (SOREMP).
Cataplexy	Loss of muscular control. Seizure-like behavior as a result of intense or sudden stimulation or emotionality. Consciousness is retained. Episodes include falling down.
Sleep Paralysis	Muscular paralysis when awakening or falling asleep.
Hypnagogic Hallucinations	Vivid dream state usually occurring during sleep paralysis, so that, because the dreamer is partially conscious, it is difficult to distinguish the dream from reality.
Associated Secondary Symptoms	
Automatic Behavior	The performance of any number of routine activities in the absence of consciousness. Resembles fugue or dissociated state with amnesia for activity.
Somnambulism	Sleep walking.
Diplopia	Altered color vision.
Nocturnal myoclonus	Violent leg jerks.
Insomnia	The inability to sleep.
Proposed Major Causative Problem	
Nocturnal disruption of sleep	Severe nightime sleep disturbance.

the experience of the hallucination is frequently not attributed to dreaming. The person may believe that the hallucinatory scenario actually took place. An associated but secondary fifth symptom is *automatic behavior* and basically consists of a lapse in consciousness while any number of routine activities are being performed.

The definition of true and total narcolepsy is composed of the four primary symptoms. A polysomnogram test, to be discussed in a later chapter, confirms the diagnosis on a physiological level. Table 2.1 presents a synopsis of the narcoleptic syndrome.

It is only in recent years that organizations have formed, such as the Narcolepsy and Cataplexy Foundation of America in New York City and the American Narcolepsy Association in San Francisco, to disseminate information about this disorder and to act as central information and research repositories. In 1975 the Montpellier conference on narcolepsy established the criteria for this diagnosis and in the same year the Association of Sleep Disorders Centers was formed.

In the following sections, basic narcoleptic symptoms will be described and analyzed with respect to their appearance, treatment, and control. It is first necessary, however, to understand normal sleeping in order to appreciate the disordered narcoleptic sleep pattern.

WHAT IS NORMAL PHYSIOLOGICAL SLEEP?

Basically, there are two kinds of sleep. One is called Rapid Eye Movement (REM) sleep, during which a person shows rapid eye movements. The eyelids will move as though the person were watching a movie while sleeping. Anyone who is awakened during REM periods will usually be able to report a dream; that is, the rapid eye movements of watching the dream may resemble the same kind of eye movements that occur while watching a movie.

REM sleep was first discovered in 1952 by Eugene Aserinsky, a graduate student who was monitoring a sleep experiment (Aserinsky and Kleitman, 1953) in the laboratory of Nathaniel Kleitman at the University of Chicago. William Dement was also working on the experiment. In 1962 Dement, Fisher and Rechtschaffen discovered the special pattern of REM sleep onset in narcoleptics (Dement, 1965; Rechtschaffen, Wolpert and Dement, 1963). Both these discoveries transformed the understanding of narcolepsy etiology from a psychological basis to a physiological or neurophysiological one. The diagnosis of narcolepsy thus became consolidated when an abnormality of REM sleep appeared on polysomnographic or brain wave testing. This kind of testing records EEG or electroencephalographic activity (brain activity), EOG or electrooculographic activity (eye movement), and EMG or electromyographic activity (muscular activity). In narcoleptics the three kinds of activity occur out of synchronization.

REM is actually correlated to a whole set of physiological activities, including inhibited or paralyzed movement, dreaming, changes in blood pressure and heart rate, and high brain activity. Dement (1972) indicates that without the muscle inhibition accompanying REM dreaming, individuals would be constantly leaping out of bed because of this high brain activity—a view not unlike the one proposed by Freud (1900), who held that people cannot move when they dream so that they are protected from acting out their aggressive impulses. Dreaming, according to Freud, also serves the purpose of permitting one to express aggression symbolically but not actually.

There are many other published studies on the nature of REM sleep. Among them are studies of the direct correspondence between eye movement and dream activity (Dement and Kleitman, 1957); the effect of rapid eye movement on cortical homeostasis (Ephron and Carrington, 1966); and a survey on basic developments in the mechanisms of sleep (Dement and Mitler, 1973).

The other type of sleep is Non-rapid Eye Movement sleep (NREM) or a non-dream sleep. Usually, NREM sleep occurs first; then, about one hour to one and a half hours later, REM or dreaming sleep begins. The two types of sleep then continue to follow each other throughout the night (Aserinsky and Kleitman, 1953). Most people spend about 20 percent of their sleep in REM or dream sleep. Approximately each 90 minutes, another REM dream period will begin. Anyone who sleeps six to eight hours per night is likely to have approximately three to five dreams.

The NREM sleep is composed of four stages. The first stage is a light sleep lasting about ten minutes. It leads into the second stage of sleep which is somewhat deeper and lasts about 30 minutes. Stage 3 sleep is deeper still and it soon leads to the deepest level of sleep called stage 4 or *D*-sleep. *D*-sleep is called *the bottom*.

As the sleeper emerges from stage 4 sleep or *D*-sleep, the REM dream period begins. A dream can last five minutes or 20 minutes. It should be stressed, however, that normal sleeping starts with NREM non-dreaming stages, and only after some time will the sleeper develop a dream. The cycle of NREM periods and REM periods then continues throughout the night. Healthy physiological sleep, therefore, is the appearance of a normal sequence of sleep cycles. Four or five of these cycles are normally experienced.

Figure 2.1 shows a typical NREM and REM chart.

THE REM RUNAWAY OF NARCOLEPSY

What happens in narcolepsy is that the narcoleptic sleep attack immediately produces a dream (Vogel, 1960). The acronym for this acute dream onset is SOREMP for Sleep Onset REM Period. As a matter of fact, the narcoleptic sleep attack is very likely designed to permit the dream to emerge. If a narcoleptic person is awakened during the sleep attack, this person will report that a dream was occurring at the moment of the attack. The simultaneous appearance of a sleep attack and the emergence of a dream will occur in the vast majority of narcoleptic cases. Many researchers of sleep disorders would describe narcolepsy as a sleep-dream onset problem (Rechtschaffen, Wolpert, Dement, et al., 1963). One way of determining whether an excessive sleeper is narcoleptic is to awaken this person at the first sign of falling asleep and ask whether a dream was occurring. If no dream is reported, then narcolepsy may in all likelihood be excluded as a possible diagnosis.

FIGURE 2.1

Sequences of States and Stages of Sleep on a Typical Night

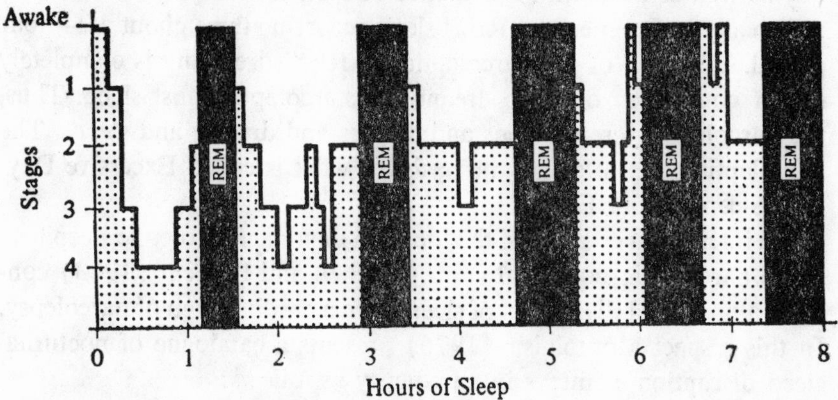

This figure is a plot of REM sleep, NREM sleep, and the four stages of NREM sleep over the course of one entire night of sleep. Although it is a "real" night from one particular subject, it is also a representative night. In other words, with a few minor changes, most nights of most people would show the identical sequence of events. The time spent in NREM sleep is lightly shaded and the time spent in REM sleep is shown in black. NREM sleep always is the first to occur at the beginning of the night. It is abnormal to go from daytime wakefulness directly into REM sleep. The first period of NREM sleep usually lasts about an hour and then gives way to the first period of REM sleep. From the onset of sleep to the end of the first REM period is the first *sleep cycle*. From the end of the first REM period to the end of the second REM period is the second sleep cycle, and so on. Thus, the cyclic alternation of NREM and REM sleep is what constitutes the basic sleep cycle that is often referred to in the literature. The average periodicity of this cycle is ninety minutes, although individual cycles may show considerable variation in length. The first sleep cycle is usually somewhat short, about seventy to eighty minutes; the second and third are usually longer than average, 100 to 110 minutes; later cycles tend to be a little shorter.

As you can see, Stages 3 and 4 dominate the NREM periods in the first part of the night, but are completely absent during the later cycles. Thus, we say that sleep is deepest in the first third of the night because we feel that it is harder to wake people up from Stage 4 sleep. The amount of Stage 2 sleep becomes progressively greater as the night wears on until it completely occupies the NREM periods toward the end of the night. The first REM period is usually relatively short, five to ten minutes, but tends to lengthen in successive cycles. Here again, individual REM periods show great variability in length, although the overall average is about twenty-two minutes. Toward the end of the night, very brief periods of wakefulness may interrupt sleep. This happens to each of us nearly every night although we may never even notice the little awakenings. In this example of an entire night, the brief periods of wakefulness were in NREM sleep, but short awakenings often occur in REM sleep as well. (From: Dement, W. C. *Some must watch while some must sleep*. San Francisco: W. H. Freeman Co., 1972).

NOCTURNAL DISRUPTION OF SLEEP

Narcoleptic people may have scores of sleep attacks throughout the day as well as at night. As a matter of fact, narcoleptic sleep attacks may really be fragments of REM sleep occurring throughout a 24-hour period. The need of the narcoleptic for REM dreaming is completely out of control; in order to dream, the narcoleptic must sleep. Thus, the narcoleptic person sleeps and dreams and dreams and sleeps. The narcoleptic sleep attack is the basis for what is called Excessive Daytime Sleepiness, or E.D.S.

An interesting contrast to the focus on daytime narcoleptic sleepiness is the narcoleptic nocturnal sleep. Mitchell and Dement (1968) consider a nocturnal disruption of sleep to be a cardinal sign of narcolepsy. In this respect Montplaisir (1976) presents a catalogue of nocturnal sleep disruption elements in narcolepsy as follows:

1. shorter sleep latency
2. more stage 1 sleep (time and percentage)
3. less stage 3 and 4 (time and percentage)
4. normal stage REM (time and percentage)
5. more body movements (mainly during REM sleep)
6. sleep onset REM periods (SOREMP—49% of recordings)
7. fragmentation of REM sleep (toward end of night)
8. alteration of the REM-NREM periodicity
9. presence of dissociated sleep
10. high incidence of frightening dreams.

Mitchell and Dement (1968) report that 85% of narcoleptic subjects have a history of severe nightime sleep disturbance. A new and hopeful treatment for narcolepsy (Gamma-Hydroxy-Butyrate) has the effect of regularizing the nocturnal sleep of narcoleptic persons, thus reducing many of the narcoleptic daytime symptoms. This point will be further discussed in Chapter 8 on the use of pharmacological agents in the treatment of narcolepsy.

THE NARCOLEPTIC SLEEP ATTACK

Most researchers would agree that the entire narcoleptic problem is genetic in origin (Kessler, 1976; Roberts, 1970; Yoss and Daly,

1960); as narcolepsy is further discussed, the biological basis of this disorder will become more evident. Several studies also have been published that indicate a predisposition for narcolepsy in some families (Daly and Yoss, 1959; Krabbe and Magnussen, 1942; Sours, 1963). There are others who discuss possible emotional and psychological bases for narcolepsy (Coodley, 1948; Missriegler, 1941; Mitchell, Dement and Gulevich, 1966; and, Szatmari and Hache, 1962). The extent to which narcolepsy is caused by biological or psychological factors will be discussed in Chapter 5.

The actual narcoleptic sleep in which REM-dream sleep begins to drag a person into a sleep drunkenness is present in almost all narcoleptic cases. This occurs even though some of the other symptoms of this disorder, such as cataplexy or sleep paralysis, may not be present. The sleep attack proper, however, is crucial to the diagnosis of narcolepsy.

Most sleep researchers are beginning to agree that narcolepsy, in the form of these classic sleep attacks, usually begins sometime in puberty, although its onset may occur even into the early 30s (Karacan, Moore and Williams, 1979). The actual narcoleptic sleep attack may be the first symptom that introduces this disorder into a person's life. In rarer cases, a cataplectic attack, in which loss of muscle control is experienced, may predate the onset of actual narcoleptic sleep attacks. Approximately 80 percent of all narcolepsy will occur before the age of 30 and the vast majority of cases will occur in males (Dement, Carskadon and Ley, 1973; Kessler, 1976); narcolepsy will appear four times more in males than in females.

Boredom, monotony and the feeling of loneliness or isolation will usually trigger a sleep attack in the narcoleptic person. For example, having to focus on one object for a long period of time can produce an element of monotony in the narcoleptic and this will begin to generate REM dream sleep. For this reason, any narcoleptic person who drives a moving vehicle is a danger to self as well as to others. It should be remembered that most narcoleptic persons, in spite of repeated failures to resist these sleep attacks, persistently cling to the idea that they will be able to successfully inhibit such attacks. This is purely wishful thinking. Sleep attacks cannot be easily inhibited and those narcoleptics who drive automobiles, will surely, at some time, be involved in accidents caused either by drowsiness or by actually falling asleep at the wheel. This issue has also been discussed by Broughton and Ghanem (1976) who present statistics on the correlation of accidents to the narcoleptic syndrome.

The narcoleptic sleep attack, although apparently organically caused, does indeed contain psychological aspects, especially with regard to those pivotal events or circumstances that stimulate the attack.

> Paul, a narcoleptic patient in his late 30s, who was attending group therapy sessions, could remain awake and alert throughout the one-and-a-half hour meeting, provided that most of the person-to-person interaction either centered around him or included him, even if in a peripheral way. If, however, the group session was one in which other members were describing events in their lives not immediately relevant to the current group situation, or if other group members were ignoring him while talking to each other, Paul would almost instantly begin to show the sleep drunkenness so characteristic of the onset of a REM dream sleep. Of course, he could quite quickly discern the extent to which any of the group interactions would be easy for him to join and this perception determined whether a sleep attack would emerge. If he sensed that he could be part of the discussion, he would remain awake and alert. If, on the other hand, he sensed that it would be difficult to join the interactions, then he would withdraw. His withdrawal would set the stage for a sleep attack to occur.

One of Paul's major personality features was a kind of inertness or passivity. It was very difficult for him to interrupt anyone actively engaged in conversation or to intervene with some personal comment when not directly involved in an ongoing interaction between other members. This personality feature is frequently associated with the one previously described in which a narcoleptic person walked 100 city blocks because he could not ask a stranger a simple question about directions. This feature of personality may also be considered as shyness, awkwardness or even fearfulness.

These may all be apt descriptions of this narcoleptic patient's inertness. However, the main point about this type of passivity and inertness is that it reveals a serious immaturity in social interactional skills. This immaturity is in direct correlation to severe dependency features in Paul's personality. When group members would focus on him, he would be happy and energized. Basically, his dependency needs were being gratified when he believed the group accepted him. This meant that other people cared about him and the interest shown by group members signalled that he could rely on them for overall emotional support and stimulation. When group members were occupied with interactions other than those focusing on him, he reported feeling profoundly cut-off and *separate*. Any time Paul felt *separated,* he would begin to experience the irresistible pull of the narcoleptic sleep attack.

This phenomenon illustrates a main point with respect to the key triggering mechanism frequently occurring in the narcoleptic sleep attack— that a profound sense of separateness can generate the attack. Thus, it may be that the monotony and boredom of driving a car at night on a straight long road causes the sleep attack for two reasons. First, the hypnotic effect of the boredom triggers a specific biological sleep reaction, and second, the experience of boredom and monotony may signal a sense of separateness.

There may be a symbolic psychological meaning to boredom. Even if a narcoleptic person is accompanied by someone, the likelihood is that boredom can still cause sleep attacks because, symbolically, it has assumed the meaning of impermanence of attachment. Such a narcoleptic person may feel that the need for dependency or attachment to another person is not being fulfilled; therefore a sense of separation anxiety can generate withdrawal reactions—the need to sleep.

Correspondingly, narcoleptic persons may undermine any sleep attack provided they feel that they are part of an ongoing stimulating interaction. In highly dependent persons with narcolepsy, however, access to social interaction will require outside help. Control over the sleep attack can be accomplished whenever a social interaction in which such a narcoleptic person participates is one that relieves separation anxiety. This means that people who are narcoleptic will probably not experience sleep attacks (or very few of these) when they are assertive and involved in some social interaction. For example, during individual psychotherapy sessions, narcoleptic patients are almost never subject to sleep attacks because the person-to-person focus is entirely on them. However, should such a person suddenly develop an attack, then it surely would be caused by some negative feelings toward the therapist that are being suppressed but which contain elements of *separateness.*

The treatment for the narcoleptic person is not, however, necessarily to create endless participatory social situations. The psychological treatment for control over the sleep attack concerns the development of a capacity for the narcoleptic person to become self-motivating, to be able to interrupt interactions when feeling excluded, and to generally increase the ability to confront other people with one's needs. This personality feature will be described in greater detail throughout the book with respect to self-corrective and psychotherapeutic treatment aims.

Narcoleptic sleep attacks can occur in the strangest ways. They are more likely to occur when the person is sitting or reclining. However, they have also been reported to have occurred while the individual was walking, so that the net result of such an attack is sleepwalking or somnambulism. Frequently, the narcoleptic person will not remember the sleep attack because it does not contain normal sleeping cues. An example of a normal sleeping cue is falling asleep into a NREM (non-dream) state and then, only after some time has elapsed, to develop dreams. The narcoleptic sleep attack produces an immediate dream and thus lacks this normal NREM cue. Upon awakening, the narcoleptic sometimes does not remember even sleeping. From time to time, the narcoleptic person will report suddenly feeling refreshed but will deny having fallen asleep. At other times, upon awakening, such persons may feel depressed, but still not believe they were asleep. Any mood that exists upon awakening may depend upon the particular personality type of the narcoleptic person. More likely it will depend upon what sort of dream was produced during the sleep attack. If the dream was particularly interesting and happy, the post-dream mood may be positive. If the dream was disturbing, then the post-dream mood may be a depressive one.

In one case, a narcoleptic person fell asleep while sitting in a chair typing a letter. Upon awakening, this person just continued typing with only a vague awareness of the intervening three or four minutes. Sometimes, while in conversation with another person, if the narcoleptic person does not really want to continue the conversation but is unable to end it, a drowsiness may suddenly appear that leads directly to a sleep attack. A narcoleptic person can even fall asleep in the midst of a sentence—much to the consternation of the listener. This behavior raises an interesting and important question about the direct expression of emotions in narcoleptic persons.

THE SPECIAL PROBLEM OF ANGER

As mentioned earlier, dependent narcoleptic persons frequently find it difficult to be direct with their feelings. This means that the dissatisfactions of such a person cannot be easily expressed. Emotions such as irritation, annoyance, anger, and especially rage generally cannot be directly ventilated. This also means that the narcoleptic person who is passive and immature expresses angry feelings and general feelings of dissatisfaction quite indirectly. What typically occurs is that a style of sarcasm is developed as a means of expressing anger. What the sarcasm does, however, is to translate angry feelings into pure hostility. In most cases, the crucial personality feature of the narcoleptic from which most of these difficulties arise is a pervasive dependency feeling. This means that many such people are quite intimidated by anyone in authority or whom they perceive to be in authority.

Narcoleptic persons who are dependent or socially immature will, in many cases, be unable to express needs directly because they usually feel unjustified in having these needs in the first place. This feeling of lack of justification stems from a sense of immaturity. The adage that children should be seen and not heard is perfectly apt in describing how this kind of person feels in relation to the rest of the world. It is the simple need of wanting to be included in a conversation, of saying something even if it means interfering in someone else's conversation, of requesting special vacation or sick leave on a job, and so forth, that this kind of person finds almost impossible to express. The idea of becoming directly angry or of expressing personal dissatisfactions directly is usually seen to be a difficult, if not impossible, task for many individuals who are severely dependent and who have narcolepsy. This is especially true because of the narcoleptic person's complicated symptom picture and the effect of cataplexy on any intense vocal disagreement. This point will be discussed in the next chapter.

Because of the dependency feelings and social fears that this kind of narcoleptic person may experience, the emotions of timidity, fear and apprehension govern behavior more than feelings of anger or dissatisfaction. The problem is that when such individuals feel angry, they either suppress it or become, as previously indicated, facetious or mainly sarcastic—indirect ways of expressing dissatisfaction. The effect of not expressing anger or dissatisfaction directly is that undue emotional restriction tends to increase the probability of a sleep attack. Frustration and anger that are withheld rather than expressed constitute major causes of the narcoleptic sleep attack. Yet, as an exception to this rule, narcoleptic persons will almost universally lose control and become angry at people who criticize them for being "lazy"—a mistaken perception created by the sleep attacks of the narcoleptic.

CONTROL OF THE NARCOLEPTIC SLEEP ATTACK

One of the psychological principles of personality dynamics about which most psychoanalysts would agree is that dependency feelings generate anger and that the more pervasive the dependency, the more pervasive the anger. Apparently, even though dependent people seek others to be dependent upon, and, in fact, wish for dependency satisfaction, they paradoxically also resent needing to depend. They really resent their immaturity. The gratification of dependency needs generates feelings of emotional security. Yet, each of these dependency gratifications eliminates the possibility of independent thought and behavior on the part of the dependent person, who intuitively realizes this. The fact that held-in dissatisfactions may be one of the main causative features of such a person's sleep attack reveals just how difficult it is for this kind of person to try to overcome the attack. How is it possible to overcome a sleep attack when it means expressing oneself in a way that is impossible to do?

Thus, those narcoleptic individuals who are emotionally and psychologically dependent may exist in a state of perpetual anger-inhibition; overcoming a sleep attack is not a simple matter. First, the source of the anger needs to be known; second, any dependency needs that were frustrated, that may have caused the anger in the first place, also need to be known. If the narcoleptic person is aware of these circumstances, then the probability of overcoming the sleep attack increases.

Of course, any resolution of severe dependency needs will always decrease the level of anger in a person. A major treatment aim for dependent persons with narcolepsy, therefore, should be to reduce dependency needs and to increase self-expression and assertiveness. Whether or not narcoleptic sleep attacks can be entirely eliminated in this fashion is highly debatable. Organic factors do seem to play the major role in narcolepsy. In psychotherapy, the analysis of dependency features of personality, however, may contribute a significant measure of control over the sleep attack because overall anger and dissatisfaction in the personality will correspondingly subside. In addition, associated with the working-out of neurotic dependency is a corresponding gradual increase in maturity level so that a more direct and face-to-face expression of emotions is possible.

The following clinical illustration shows improvement in the narcoleptic sleep attack based upon therapeutic gains that are characterized by a greater ability to express feelings directly.

> Mark, a 35-year-old engineer who would frequently fall asleep at his drafting table began to repeat this behavior in the therapy group. He could not easily join in any interaction and he would wait to be approached by other group members. Whenever he was invited into an interaction, he greatly appreciated the opportunity to participate. Such invitations satisfied his dependency needs

because he could not, on his own, enter into the proceedings. When he was not focused upon, or, when he allowed a large amount of group time to elapse without participating, he would become angry but would not express his anger. Invariably, he would begin to develop a sleep attack. He could not avoid it. When other group members would say his name or touch his hand or knee, he would awaken just as suddenly as he fell asleep.

After some months, Mark began handling his conflicts better and began to resolve some of his problems. He learned to become more direct and less intimidated. He actually became less dependent, felt more mature, and was not as angry about his incapacities. His sleep attacks in the group dramatically decreased because he was involved in many more interactions—frequently without waiting for invitations to participate.

Mark's problem of narcolepsy began, when he was 18, with a sudden irresistible urge to sleep. He left home to attend college and the leaving set off a separation reaction—in this case, a narcoleptic symptom. This school housed students in individual homes surrounding the campus, and Mark's room was in one of these homes. The house had a *separate* entrance from the street. Mark was a bright student, but had also been extremely dependent upon his parents throughout his growing-up years. He was always obedient, never expressed the open defiance and rebelliousness typically seen during adolescence, and was somewhat on the periphery of all of his social circles. Upon entering college, he felt an overwhelming homesickness that especially bothered him when he was alone in his rented room. The therapy sessions helped Mark gain a measure of maturity and his sarcasm and overall indirectness lessened. He was extremely relieved to gain some measure of control over his sleep attack. He was also more consistent in maintaining his medication regimen in contrast to his previous behavior when he would often neglect to take his medication regularly.

SUMMARY

In this chapter, the first and most telling symptom of the narcoleptic problem—the narcoleptic sleep attack itself—was analyzed with respect to its onset, its debilitating effects, its emotional properties, and its potential response to therapeutic intervention. The narcoleptic sleep attack is an organic biological problem that has psychological and emotional aspects. It is these psychological features that may be addressed psychotherapeutically so that they can be minimized. Psychotherapy alone cannot eliminate narcoleptic sleep attacks. However, psychotherapy can help the narcoleptic person resolve personality conflicts such as those involving the severe dependency-separation experience, the problem of the inability to express dissatisfactions, and the overall social-maturity problem. These treatment goals are well worth working for.

In the next chapter, the second major narcoleptic symptom—the cataplexy—will be described with respect to onset of attacks, effects of the attacks, special problems they make for the narcoleptic person, and how such cataplectic attacks may be treated psychotherapeutically so that they, too, may be better controlled.

Chapter 3

Cataplexy: The Losing Control Problem

WHAT IS CATAPLEXY?

Cataplexy was described earlier as a loss of muscle tone. The cataplectic attack causes the narcoleptic person to lose control over all voluntary muscles. Weakness may occur in isolated muscle groups such as in the jaw, in head dropping, or in facial sagging. When the cataplectic attack occurs, a person may simply fall down. In the early 1900s, the term cataplexy was first used to mean a temporary muscle tonelessness caused by the expression of *sudden* emotionality and accompanied by a transitory paralysis. This definition of cataplexy is still accurate. The main point about the motor paralysis is that it occurs instantaneously and passes after a few minutes.

Cataplexy literally means being struck down. The attack may last a few seconds, and in some instances it may last for five or ten minutes. During the cataplectic attack, consciousness is not lost even while the subject is in a collapsed condition. There is no feeling of having been asleep, and hearing and other senses remain generally intact, although space orientation for limb position may be lost. Most importantly, the cataplectic person mostly remains consistently in touch with reality. Thus, in the vast majority of cases, nothing else occurs other than the experience of collapsing. The general cataplectic symptom is described in Guilleminault (1976) and in Karacan, Moore and Williams (1979). An example of this kind of experience was described by Paul —a patient cited in the previous chapter.

> I was having dinner with my family—my wife, mother, father and sister. My sister said something funny at which the entire family, in unison, burst into loud laughter. It was like a bolt of lightening hitting me when I first heard the joke and the collective shot of laughter. I instantly fell off my chair onto the floor. I could feel my body convulsing but I was not able to do anything about it. I was completely conscious of everyone running around me. My mother told my sister to get a wet towel while my father and my wife tried to hold me and even lift me up. It was a familiar scene to everyone because it had happened so many times before —so that no one was really in any kind of panic. I recovered after about two or three minutes and raised myself to my feet. I was perfectly all right and reminded my mother, as I had so many times in the past, that cold compresses don't really help. She never seems to remember that because basically she feels she is the only one who knows how to help me.

This clinical illustration is quite typical of the cataplectic attack. These attacks are reported to be usually stimulated by great excitement or intense emotionality or sudden emotion.

Therapists and researchers have attributed the cataplectic attack to intense anger, joy, laughter, sarcasm, surprise, startle, anxiety, threat and a whole host of other intense emotions, even including despair. In Table 3.1, a list of situations that induce cataplectic attacks is provided by Guilleminault (1976).

The attacks generally follow the same pattern—that is, collapsing and losing control of voluntary muscles, being unable to control the involuntary body movements that occur during the attack, being completely conscious and simply waiting till the muscular paralysis passes. In rare instances, some narcoleptics will experience perceptual problems during the cataplectic attack. They may not be as aware; the level of consciousness in such people may indeed be reduced and individual sense organs may be affected. For example, blurred vision or hearing

TABLE 3.1

Situations That Induce Cataplexy

Number of Positive Responses (N = 130)	Situations
123	Laughter
112	Anger
91	Feeling of amusement
78	Athletic activity
75	Excitement
68	Elation
65	Resisting a sleep attack
62	Surprise
60	Tension
47	Attempt at repartee
42	Spontaneous (with no known cause)
40	Response to call for action
40	Sexual intercourse
38	Fear
36	Embarrassment
25	Swimming
10	Yawning
10	Revulsion
8	Sighing
1	Driving an automobile

Reprinted by permission from Table 1, page 129, Chapter 7 in *Narcolepsy* by Christian Guilleminault, Ed. Copyright 1976, Spectrum Publications, Inc., New York.

difficulties may occur and some numbness of limbs may be experienced. In even rarer cases, smell and taste may be affected. Upon the passing of the attack, however, these difficulties also subside and normal functioning is resumed.

This peculiar symptom formation of cataplexy raises the question of whether cataplexy is different from epilepsy. The answer to this question is that cataplexy is a distinctly different disorder. Dement (1972), a pioneer in the field of sleep research, has demonstrated that the brain activity of a narcoleptic person as measured by the electroencephalograph (EEG) is regular, whereas the brain activity of a person with epilepsy or variations of epilepsy is usually scattered or irregular. The relation of narcolepsy to the epilepsies is presented by Bonduelle and Degos (1976), Cohn and Cruvant (1944) and Tharp

(1976). It is now acknowledged by researchers that cataplexy is actually a breakthrough of the paralysis accompanying REM. It should also be noted that the term *catalepsy* (frequently confused with *cataplexy*) refers specifically to hysterical reactions occurring in conditions of schizophrenia and has nothing whatever to do with the symptom expressions of narcolepsy.

VARIATIONS IN THE OCCURRENCE OF CATAPLEXY

The onset of cataplexy is quite varied and may occur in a multitude of ways, in contrast to the onset of narcolepsy which is simply experienced as an overwhelming need to sleep. The narcoleptic sleep attack is reported by researchers to occur spontaneously without any external triggering event. However, in the previous discussion on narcoleptic sleep, it was pointed out that many kinds of situations that may cause dissatisfactions in the narcoleptic can cause sleep attacks. This is especially true since it is likely that in such persons feelings of dissatisfactions may be suppressed and thereby withdrawal into sleep can occur. Yet, the accepted view of the entire narcoleptic disorder is that the narcoleptic sleep attack occurs spontaneously while cataplexy is always caused by external events. The causes and effects of both the narcoleptic sleep attack and the cataplexy should be discerned because in 95 percent of cases when one symptom is present, so is the other (Guilleminault, 1976). Of all narcoleptics it is estimated that about 15 percent experience the entire tetrad and that generally sleep attacks predate the appearance of cataplexy by several years.

Generally, most authors would agree with Kleitman (1963) in his view that boredom and monotony cause narcolepsy while sudden excitement favors cataplexy. In a minority of cases, the cataplectic attack may even predate by several months the onset of the entire narcoleptic disorder.

There are many variations in the onset of cataplexy. These have ranged from attacks upon falling asleep to those caused by sexual excitement. Some researchers have noted that certain cataplectic attacks occurred at the onset of sleep or at the time of awakening. In such cases, attacks were accompanied by abnormal dream states or by hallucinations. This phenomenon will be reviewed and discussed in the following chapter on sleep paralysis and hypnagogic hallucinations. Farber (1962) cites a case of a narcoleptic man in whom cataplexy occurred before the narcoleptic sleep attack and before the appearance of any other narcoleptic symptom:

> "The episode started approximately at the age of 35 with a cataplectic attack after he had related something humorous to several fellow employees. It was something uncomplimentary. Then one side of his face felt numb. This was followed by tingling sensation of muscles of that side of the face also followed a few days later by a cataplectic attack. Narcolepsy appeared a few weeks later."

Morgenstern (1965) reports a case in which a cataplectic attack occurred at the moment of orgasm. The cataplexy occurred at the point of seminal emission. This sort of cataplectic attack has been called orgasmolepsie.

The overall relationship of sexual activity to motor control has been related to episodes of loss of consciousness. This was even suggested by Hippocrates, and Charcot and Freud also stated that sexual impulses affected the narcoleptic disorder.

Morgenstern further reports that one of his patients experienced cataplectic attacks in response to embarrassment or laughter. The patient reported experiencing instantaneous relaxation of all muscles beginning a week or two after the sleep symptoms. This patient had to relinquish his inclination to tease others. The effect of his teasing would evoke a loss of muscle tone. This kind of teasing is an example of the indirect expression of emotions typical of narcoleptic persons with dependency problems. Sarcasm and teasing have been reported in many other sources as triggering mechanisms of the cataplectic attack.

Gélineau, who in the late 1800s coined the term narcolepsy, also personally experienced the problem of cataplexy (Gélineau, 1880). He would, from time to time, manifest cataplectic attacks on the streets of Paris. He was, of course, completely conscious during such attacks, and at times was unable to overcome them because onlookers gathering around him would be sympathetic to his plight. Gélineau experienced an intense emotional response to their sympathy, causing even more severe and prolonged paralysis. Because of this recurring cataplexy, he could not lift himself up from the ground.

The narcoleptic person is in a dilemma. Monotony is not good because it can cause sleep attacks, yet excitement is not good because it can cause cataplexy. Narcoleptic patients sometimes feel that the only way to function is to be emotionally neutral so as to minimize recurring attacks. There are some narcoleptic individuals who have experienced 100 or more cataplectic attacks per day.

There may be some one-half million or more people in this country alone who experience this particular aspect of narcolepsy. The question that must be analyzed with respect to this seizure-like disorder refers to the specific nature of those intense emotions that can cause cataplexy. Is there anything special about such intense emotional triggering mechanisms that can offer a clue to possible psychological treatment and perhaps partial control of cataplexy?

In the following section, it will be suggested that all cataplectic attacks are triggered by the specific element of *surprise* contained in the emotional context between the narcoleptic person and whoever or whatever else is involved in any ongoing social interaction.

CATAPLEXY AND THE EMOTION OF SURPRISE

The element of surprise will almost always be the key triggering mechanism of the cataplectic attack. In Table 3.1, although Guilleminault (1976) does not attribute the emotional component of surprise as the key triggering mechanism of all cataplectic attacks, it may be seen that this emotion is present in almost all of the reactions listed. Though there is certainly no agreement among sleep researchers or writers on narcolepsy regarding a single causative agent in the onset of a cataplectic attack, except perhaps that it is caused by intense emotion (Karacan, Moore and Williams, 1979), a careful analysis of case histories perhaps can reveal that the element of surprise was present in each case. Gélineau was unable to control his attack perhaps because each time he heard a sympathetic response from an onlooker it created a personal sense between him and the sympathetic person that was, in an existential sense, startling. The unexpected element in the startle experience is equivalent to the element of surprise.

A response of surprise can produce muscular weakness in anyone; for example, people frequently are unable to run or even walk when they hear a very funny joke, especially when it makes them *convulse* with laughter. People are even heard to say something like, "It was so funny *I almost fell down* laughing." The unexpected or surprising punch-line ending to a joke is apparently a powerful agent in its effect on the brain mechanism that regulates voluntary muscles. Bonstedt (1954) discusses such brain mechanisms as well as emotional aspects of narcoleptic symptomatology, and in an early study Brock and Wiesel (1941) discuss the entire narcoleptic-cataplectic syndrome as an excessive reaction of the sleep mechanism. It should be remembered that cataplexy was first used as a term to indicate *sudden* or *surprising* emotionality. Paul's cataplectic response to a joke told at the dinner table was reinforced by the uniform and synchronous *sudden* outburst of laughter of the entire family. The collective understanding of the punch line reinforced the sense of surprise Paul himself felt about the joke and this reinforced reaction of surprise thereby intensified his attack.

In many cases, even the expression of intense anger will not cause the cataplectic attack if, in advance, the anger was anticipated. The only way in which anticipated anger can produce the cataplectic attack is if the sound of the angry outburst is itself, each time, surprising to the person expressing and then hearing it. There are those individuals who become astounded when they are able to express anger even though they may do so quite frequently. Apparently, such people view themselves as timid and "civilized"; when they become angry, it never quite sounds to them as though the anger emanates from themselves. The vocal sound of the anger is a kind of existential shock each time it occurs. This kind of shock can produce a cataplectic attack. *In such cases, the element of surprise is an effect of the anger and not the anger itself.*

Other emotions such as intense joy, laughter or sarcasm will similarly cause the cataplectic attack, but, it is suggested here, only if the element of surprise is an effect of these specific emotions. Cataplexy that appears at the onset of sleep may occur, therefore, because the moment of losing consciousness and falling into sleep implies something different that suddenly happened in an automatic manner. This automatic falling into sleep, even though it is quite natural, carries with it an implied moment of surprise at the transition point of wakefulness to sleepfulness. The cataplexy, then, is transformed into an equivalent sleep paralysis. Similarly, cataplectic attacks that occur during sexual activity are also the result of transition points from control over sexual excitement to loss of control during orgasm. With some, the mere act of sexual caressing defines this transition point. All such transition points contain an element of surprise and will evoke cataplectic reactions. In the telling of a joke, the narcoleptic person observes surprise in the facial expression of the other person at the punch line of the joke, and this alone—the identification and observation of surprise—is enough to cause a cataplectic attack. Laughter and joke-telling also have special relevance to the relation between surprise and sarcasm.

Many narcoleptic dependent individuals, as previously mentioned, find it difficult to be direct in expressing dissatisfactions or the desire to have personal needs gratified. It is not unusual for sarcastic and witty repartee to be characteristic of dependency and passivity features in the narcoleptic's personality. The problem with this style is that it is quite effective in deflating the ego of the unfortunate recipient of the witty sarcastic remark, whose facial reaction usually reveals a display of embarrassment or surprise. The observation of this facial expression can be instantly sufficient to produce a cataplectic attack in the narcoleptic.

A sarcastic style is developed out of this kind of person's inability to be direct with feelings. The use of sarcastic remarks and a general overall style of sarcasm are simply a compromise formation—a way of satisfying both sides of a conflict, such as the need to inhibit anger as well as to express it. Thus, sarcasm is a compromise formation for this kind of narcoleptic person because it is a way of being assertive, (especially in terms of expressing one's dissatisfactions) without addressing such concerns in a face-to-face, talking-it-out manner. Each sarcastic remark can cause a look of surprise in another person and, as a result, immediately generate a cataplectic attack in the narcoleptic. Thus, teasing, sarcasm and facetious behavior can and will ignite cataplectic attacks.

Those narcoleptic people who respond sarcastically—seeking always to be pungent, condescending and generally angry—can generate anywhere from 25 to 50 or more cataplectic attacks per day.

The element of surprise can cause the cataplectic attack not only when it is the narcoleptic who jokes or makes the sarcastic remark, but also when it is objectively witnessed as part of someone else's interaction.

> A narcoleptic patient could not watch a well-known comedian on television because the sort of sarcastic, biting and embarrassing humor typical of this entertainer's style would cause a major cataplectic attack in this patient. This type of severe cataplectic attack is just as often self-imposed as it is caused by external events.

There are times when the narcoleptic person will believe that the cataplectic attack occurred "out of the blue" without any cause whatsoever. It may be claimed that no other person was around, nothing really noteworthy was happening, and there were no especially loud noises by which to be surprised in the immediate environment. Yet, in such cases, careful examination of the narcoleptic person's train of thought immediately preceding the attack will more often than not reveal that a detailed scenario was occurring in this person's daydreaming. For example, a typical fantasy is one in which a triumphant moment was achieved—probably through the defeat of another person who was embarrassed by the narcoleptic person's outstandingly clever wit. The narcoleptic person is then stunned by the look of surprise in the defeated partner's facial expression and this startle can cause the cataplectic attack. Such fantasies are not unusual and occur because this type of person cannot easily express dissatisfactions directly and therefore needs to create daydreams in which anger is successfully expressed and even overemphasized. The main point to be remembered here is that the cataplectic attack always has a cause and its triggering mechanism is the emotion of surprise. This sequence of feeling surprised and then experiencing a cataplectic attack may occur in actual social interaction or it may just as easily occur as a result of a fantasy.

TREATMENT AND CONTROL OF CATAPLEXY

The cataplectic attack is most effectively controlled by the correct medication and this issue is discussed in Chapter 8. However, most narcoleptic persons try to manage or control the cataplectic attacks by using inventive techniques that address the issue of muscular control—that is, most narcoleptic persons will try to control a cataplectic attack immediately as it begins. A typical technique is to try to clench onto something. Since the cataplectic attack causes loss of muscle tone, then it would seem quite natural for a person in the grip of such an attack to try to maintain effective muscle tone. Actually, the attempt to try to clench onto something is quite a good idea. It is partially successful in shortening the duration of the attack and in some cases is successful in short-circuiting it entirely.

Of course, the most effective way to control cataplectic attacks is to help the narcoleptic person modify certain basic personality inclinations. For example, the dependent person with narcolepsy who may need to be sarcastic because of an inability to be direct can become more direct and assertive and this goal can be addressed as a short-term psychotherapy aim. This psychological and emotional issue needs to be treated both with respect to the general narcoleptic sleep attack and in terms of cataplectic attacks. When narcoleptic persons with these particular personality conflicts can be straightforward in trying to satisfy their own needs and in the more direct expression of frustrations and dissatisfactions, then the tendency toward the use of sarcasm may become less necessary.

> When Mark first entered treatment he was unable to say anything that was free from a kind of self-aggrandizing wisdom. He

> was always trying to be clever. He was very sarcastic and could not be simple and direct with anyone. As a result, he experienced at least 10-20 cataplectic attacks per day which were triggered by the effects of his sarcastic style.
>
> Mark's major therapeutic gain was that he actually learned not to seek the pun, not to speak in witty clichés, and not to seek to be condescending in all social interaction. After six months in treatment, his cataplectic attacks were reduced by half.

To work-through or to resolve feelings of inferiority, dependency needs, and separation fears will improve one's ability to be increasingly direct in person-to-person interactions. In such cases, sarcasm will subside as will the frequency of cataplectic attacks; no longer will the only armamentarium against these attacks be the attempts to clench onto something or the attempts to fall back into a chair instead of falling onto the floor in a dead heap.

Both the narcoleptic sleep attack and the cataplectic attack have been discussed in these first few chapters. In the next chapter the remaining symptoms of the narcoleptic tetrad—sleep paralysis and hypnagogic hallucinations—will be examined. In addition, other, similarly exotic sleep symptoms that appear in narcolepsy as secondary problems, such as automatic behavior, will also be described.

Chapter 4

Sleep Paralysis, Hypnagogic Hallucinations and Other Sleep Problems of Narcolepsy

WHAT IS SLEEP PARALYSIS?

Individuals with sleep paralysis may be lying in bed in a semi-conscious state, about to fall asleep, or in a state in which they are about to awaken from sleep when they suddenly realize that they are totally paralyzed. They are completely unable to move and don't know how to get out of this dilemma or whether they will, in fact, ever get out of it. Generally, however, the sleep paralysis is episodic and passes in a few minutes.

Sleep paralysis is a major symptom of narcolepsy even though not all narcoleptics experience it. Its organic basis is discussed by Brock (1944) and some chemical treatment issues are considered by Weitzner (1952). Some estimates of the occurrence of each of the four major symptoms of narcolepsy reveal that sleep paralysis itself appears in about one-quarter of all narcoleptic persons. Hishikawa (1976) reports the incidence of sleep paralysis as between 14 and 57 percent in narcoleptic patients. It is less of a problematic or debilitating symptom than cataplexy because it generally will not interfere with one's social relationships. It will usually occur at bedtime or in the morning upon awakening. If a narcoleptic person naps during the day, then it may also occur at that point.

Sleep paralysis was first identified in the last half of the 19th century. It is a paralysis that is similar to the one seen in cataplexy. However, it occurs during the period of relaxation or reduced consciousness between falling asleep and the state of sleep itself, as well as between the points of unconsciousness—when one is asleep—and semi-consciousness when one is awakening (Goode, 1962; Everett, 1963; Hishikawa, 1976; Sours, 1963). A person who frequently experiences this disorder is likely to describe it as "I wake up before my body." Apparently, the state of muscular relaxation, which exists, for example, in the process of going to sleep increases the likelihood of a sleep paralysis attack. If, during a sleep paralysis attack, some outside physical contact is made with such persons, they will awaken and again regain control of all motoric functions and of all voluntary muscles.

In sleep paralysis, the definition of REM sleep is not conventionally satisfied; a suppression of muscle activity occurs, but the REM pattern and the low voltage frequency pattern in the EEG are atypical. In addition, the three are unsynchronized. The sleep paralysis occurs as a "breakthrough" phenomenon: when the person is awake the phenomenon occurs as a cataplectic attack, but during the awakening from sleep or going to sleep it emerges as the sleep paralysis.

Sleep paralysis also afflicts people who are not narcoleptic. When the sleep-paralysis attack occurs in non-narcoleptic persons, there are sure to be emotional problems that contribute to the development of such symptoms (Everett, 1963; Schneck, 1969).

> A striking example of sleep paralysis in a non-narcoleptic person occurred in Alvin, a man of 26 who sought psychotherapy because he was profoundly unable to express himself directly and had recently been severely embarrassed by this incapacity. He was not mute and could answer all questions asked of him, but would not reveal any of his feelings on his own. He was a very handsome young man who would, by his mere presence, attract

the attentions of women. This presented him with a problem because although he welcomed this interest, it also meant that he would have to engage in at least nominal social intercourse and he was unable to participate even in such basic interactions. He was exceedingly gracious and generous and was a genuinely nice person. He was also painfully inhibited and thus effectively incapacited.

Alvin finally sought help after meeting a young woman whom he liked but could not pursue because of his special problems. This dilemma generated his first attack of sleep-paralysis in which, upon awakening one morning. he found himself unable to move. He reported feeling completely paralyzed and became panic-stricken. During this paralysis and panic, he felt as though he was blowing up like a balloon—larger and larger—until he was so big that he was close to the ceiling of the room and, in fact, could feel that his body was filling up the entire room. As his proportions grew, his panic became mixed with a surreal quality. He was jolted out of the sleep paralysis by the simultaneous ringing of the alarm clock and by his mother who was shaking his leg.

Alvin was an extremely dependent person who lived at home with his parents, two brothers and three sisters. At home he could never do anything on his own because there was always someone to do it for him. In fact, he was, in quite an unmalicious way, encouraged not to do anything. In therapy sessions, it was soon apparent that beneath his casual appearance was a very angry person. His immediate problem was that his reservoir of anger was so great that it was literally *blowing him up* during the attack of sleep-paralysis.

Alvin wanted to move to his own apartment because he felt that he needed this sort of privacy in order to invite friends over and thus become more social. However he was still afraid to be on his own and the therapist agreed that this would be undesirable for two main reasons. The first was that he could become overly isolated in his own apartment. He was a person who had not developed even the most rudimentary social skills; he could not be direct about his feelings or his needs, and his anger about his overall dependency and incapacities was so great that it was virtually paralyzing him.

The second reason for the decision not to move to his own apartment was based upon the diagnosis of his condition. His sleep-paralysis could have been the advance warning of an emerging narcoleptic condition. If this were so, the *separation* from his parents upon whom he was so *dependent* could easily have become the triggering mechanism for the appearance of other narcoleptic symptoms or for the emergence of the entire narcoleptic problem itself.

Alvin remained at his parents' home and began psychotherapy treatment. As he described his life, he began to ventilate feelings of dissatisfaction towards many important people around him. This newfound ability to express himself soon eliminated the attacks of sleep-paralysis as well as the strange phenomenon of the feeling of blowing-up. After three months in treatment, no further narcoleptic symptoms appeared. After one year in psychotherapy treatment, the issue of leaving home was again raised. It remained a delicate issue for a while and its resolution was only gradually accomplished. Alvin made the transition when separation-anxiety problems subsided.

Alvin's sleep-paralysis is an example of the classic narcoleptic sleep-paralysis even though he had never experienced the entire narcolepsy symptom tetrad. His feeling of blowing-up resembled the narcoleptic symptom associated with sleep-paralysis called the hypnagogic hallucination. This type of hallucination will be described in the following section.

THE HYPNAGOGIC HALLUCINATION

The definition of hallucination, generally, is the seeing of something that is not there; for example, severely disturbed patients in mental hospitals who are diagnosed as having acute schizophrenia or other diagnoses of psychosis may, from time to time, report hearing voices speaking to them directly when, in reality, they may have been quite alone. Others may see some apparition such as the figure of a person looming in the distance when no such person is present. It is frequently reported that alcoholics may typically hallucinate walls full of crawling cockroaches or rats. The hypnagogic hallucination is much the same kind of perception except that it creates the vivid feeling of reality during the sleep-paralysis attack (McKellar and Simpson, 1954;

Schacter, 1976; Slight, 1924; Vihvelin, 1948). A person experiencing sleep-paralysis is in a state of decreased consciousness—either falling into sleep or emerging from it. It is at such moments that the hypnagogic hallucination will occur. Alvin would swear that he actually was blowing-up.

There are times when a narcoleptic person will experience an attack of sleep-paralysis and an accompanying hypnagogic hallucination and later, upon awakening, will not be able to tell whether the hallucination was something that actually occurred or was just a dream. The experience is so vivid that a bit of skepticism remains and one thinks that perhaps it did happen, even though the content of the hallucination may be bizarre, thereby revealing its impossible nature.

When Alvin was able to regain control over his muscles and fully awakened from the hallucination, he realized that he could not have possibly blown up to the size of his bedroom, and yet, he harbored the distinct feeling that it had happened. Obviously, this kind of hallucination gets a profound grip on one's beliefs to the extent of competing rather effectively with one's sense of reality.

THE TYPICAL NARCOLEPTIC'S HYPNAGOGIC HALLUCINATION

One of the most typical hypnagogic hallucinations experienced by narcoleptic persons involves the *intruder in the house* experience. During the attack of sleep-paralysis, the hypnagogic hallucination will involve the imagining of someone entering one's premises and either ransacking the house or simply rummaging around. In fact, the person having the sleep-paralysis will, through the hallucination, more than likely see the intruder entering the room and, with total disregard of being observed, this intruder will appear to go about doing whatever he or she came to do. In some instances, this hallucination generates fear, but more often it is just observed in a detached way.

> Mark would hallucinate *the intruder* whenever he had a sleep-attack. The intruder was always the same man—the janitor of the building. He would enter Mark's bedroom and, while disregarding Mark, proceed to rummage around the room even to the point

of searching near the bed where Mark was lying. At times, their heads would almost touch. Mark, therefore, lying there paralyzed, was seeing this other man, at times, no further than a few inches from him. It is no wonder that upon awakening he could not believe it was simply a dream he had been having. After such experiences, whenever Mark actually saw the janitor it would make him feel peculiar. He was never able to convince himself that it had not really happened.

The similarity of the hypnagogic hallucination to an anxiety dream or to a nightmare has been noticed by many therapists. There are also studies to show that the hypnagogic hallucination occurs during REM dream sleep. Apparently, the sleep-paralysis is accompanied by the onset of a dream and the hypnagogic hallucination may be part of the dream process or the dream itself. Some believe that the hypnagogic hallucination is a nightmare, in contrast to conventional non-nightmare dreams. Ernest Jones (1949) has discussed the comparison between the hypnagogic hallucination and the nightmare. He states that the common ingredient between both states is the ever-present helpless paralysis. A discussion of sleep paralysis, hypnagogic hallucinations and their relationship to the nightmare is presented by Liddon (1967). There are also special hypnagogic hallucinations with dangerous implications.

A narcoleptic patient reported one such hypnagogic hallucination that occurred while he was driving an automobile at night. He suddenly hallucinated someone walking in front of the car. He swerved the car and almost experienced a cataplectic attack because of his momentary *surprise*. The cataplectic attack never materialized because he was already clenching onto the wheel and the clenching experience enabled him to gain control over his muscles.

The hallucinated figure that *suddenly* walked in front of the car apparently was a variation of the *intruder* theme and strongly suggests that the experience of driving an automobile in a relaxed state can generate cataplectic or sleep paralysis attacks along with accompanying hypnagogic hallucinations. Other typical hypnagogic hallucinations include: floating, out of body experiences, and even flying.

This variation in the usual appearance of hypnagogic hallucinations also points out that the narcoleptic syndrome consists of many kinds of sleep disturbance problems. These are discussed in the following section.

OTHER NARCOLEPTIC SLEEP SYMPTOMS

When a narcoleptic person shows the entire narcoleptic tetrad—the narcoleptic sleep attack, cataplexy, sleep paralysis and hypnagogic hallucinations—it is highly likely that a multitude of other sleep anomalies will also be experienced. Among these additional sleep problems are: fugue or dissociated states with amnesia, somnambulism or sleepwalking, various forms of insomnia (due to excessive sleeping periods throughout the day), diplopia or altered color vision, and nocturnal myoclonus or violent leg jerks that may occur during sleep throughout the night (see Table 1.1).

> Mark experienced frequent fugue or automatic behavior states. He would continue to do whatever he was doing at any given time but would have total amnesia for the period of time in the fugue state. He once reported an extremely interesting incident in which he remembers beginning to take a final examination only to find himself walking home. He remembered going to class and beginning to take the exam. He did not remember finishing it or submitting his exam paper or leaving the room or leaving the campus. He immediately returned to class, located his instructor and checked to see whether, in fact, he had submitted his paper. His instructor produced the examination paper. It was completely finished but somewhat jumbled. The instructor said that Mark had smiled when submitting his paper and then just walked out like any other student.

Researchers believe that 10 to 15 percent of all narcoleptic people experience automatic behavior. A frequent fugue or automatic state experienced by Mark, who worked in an engineering firm, occurred when he was walking from his drafting table to the far side of the room. Almost every day when he would do this, he would find himself back at his desk with no memory of having walked across the room.

> In the therapy sessions, this behavior was considered in terms of why it occurred only under those circumstances. Mark was asked to describe the physical location of objects and of people who worked with him in the office. The assumption was that something interpersonal was causing this particular automatic behavior and that the fugue itself may have been Mark's indirect expression of anger or embarrassment or some other feeling toward a specific person. Upon hearing this, Mark announced that he had an enormous crush on Sally, an engineering associate who had joined the firm six months before. It became clear that this feeling toward Sally was in some way probably responsible for Mark's fugues, especially since, to his best recollection, he had never experienced these particular dissociated episodes before Sally arrived on the scene.
>
> Mark then changed his route in the office to avoid Sally. It was only after she began talking to him about work-related matters that he became less awestruck with her. She was friendly to him and he could feel that he had access to her. They became office chums, and Sally would freely discuss her boyfriend and her personal life. Mark actually told her he liked her very much and she responded by saying she was flattered.
>
> Following these developments, Mark worked during therapy sessions on his ability to simply say what was on his mind within reasonable social limits. As his feelings for Sally gained realistic proportions, he was less frightened of her and less angry about his incapacity to reach out to her, as had previously been the case. The automatic behavior gradually subsided until it almost entirely disappeared. Mark worked at this job for three years after his episodes subsided and they did not recur with respect to Sally, although he occasionally displayed such behavior with respect to other activities.

Thus, with regard to the control of the automatic behavior episodes, a psychotherapeutic intervention helped Mark improve certain psychological and emotional problems so that the effects of these problems (the appearance of fugue or dissociated or automatic behavior) could be minimized.

It is interesting to see how many of the narcoleptic symptoms are paradoxically caused; for example, monotony helps reduce cataplexy but it will trigger a narcoleptic sleep attack. On the other hand, excitement is good for avoiding a narcoleptic sleep attack but it can cause a cataplectic attack. Similarly, somnambulism, which is a fugue-like state while asleep, reflects a set of causal conditions opposite to those causing cataplexy and sleep-paralysis. In cataplexy and in sleep paralysis, the mind seems to be conscious and alert, or in some way in touch with reality, and yet muscular and motoric capacities are quite asleep. In somnambulism, the mind seems to be unconscious and asleep or in some other way anesthetized and yet muscular and motoric capacities are quite awake.

Sleepwalking or somnambulism is, of course, quite dangerous. It is apparent that the entire narcoleptic disorder creates tremendous problems for anyone who has it. Narcoleptic persons may be dismissed from one job after another because of falling asleep at their desks. They may be found lying on the floor in a state of cataplexy. They may be found walking in a fugue-like way displaying automatic behavior around the office. At night while sleepwalking they can cause accidents that are quite harmful. Bouts of sleep-paralysis are also troublesome for the narcoleptic and the appearance of hypnagogic hallucinations can cause accidents while driving any kind of moving vehicle. As indicated earlier, swerving a car while driving because of a hallucination in which a person is seen walking in front of the car is not an uncommon experience during a brief sleep-paralysis.

There are many other minor variations of sleep problems experienced by the narcoleptic (Roth, 1978). They range from diplopia or altered color vision—a precursor of cataplexy—to various forms of wakefulness at night. Discussion of some of these insomnia symptoms will be found in the chapters on insomnia.

The issue of the extent to which narcolepsy is a physical-organic disorder or the result of a psychological-emotional conflict is the subject of a number of theories. Most researchers now agree that narcolepsy is a neurophysiological disorder. Yet some psychotherapeutic intervention can be successful in decreasing narcoleptic symptoms. Based upon the evidence so far compiled by researchers of sleep problems, by psychopharmacologists and by psychotherapists, it is clear that this disorder does indeed have an organic-physiological basis, and that, unquestionably, an entire psychological-emotional superstructure is imposed onto the biological problem.

The psychological treatment of narcolepsy can minimize many of the narcoleptic symptoms but it cannot eliminate narcolepsy. Whether or not psychopharmacological treatment can eliminate it, given the disorder's psychological and emotional counterparts, is at this time a debatable question. In the following chapter some of the biological and psychological theories of narcolepsy will be presented.

Chapter 5

Biological and Psychological Theories of Narcolepsy

A BIOLOGICAL BASIS FOR NARCOLEPSY

Research into the organic basis for narcolepsy has suggested a whole host of possible physical causes for this disorder. Some investigators have proposed that narcolepsy is a genetic disorder, handed down in families the way any genetic disorder is transmitted (Leckman and Gershon, 1976; Kessler, 1976; Krabbe and Magnussen, 1942; Yoss and Daly, 1960). Sours (1963) reports that, in a study of 115 cases, 12 to 33 percent of all narcoleptic subjects had a positive history of the disorder in their families. In addition, Daly and Yoss (1959) studied one family generationally and found that 13 different members (plus three suspected) over four generations had narcolepsy. Along with this finding, research is developing showing the inheritability of sleep patterns among different species (Prudom and Klemm, 1973; Van Twyver, 1969; Zung and Wilson, 1967), and the genetic transmission of narcolepsy and cataplexy even in strains of dogs (Mitler, 1976).

The variety of physical causes attributed to the onset of narcolepsy have ranged from specific trauma to the brain, as occurs, for example, in a bad fall, to endocrine dysfunction or a dysfunction of hormonal secretions, severe infections, epilepsy, tumors of the brain, and skin and circulatory disturbances. Some of these issues are discussed in Kales (1969), Lugaresi (1961), Rechtschaffen and Dement (1967), Roberts (1970), and Roth, Bruhova and Lehovsky (1968). The issue of narcoleptic symptomatology as a result of injury or reduction of cortical activity is also reported in Ethelberg (1950, 1956) and Szatmari and Hache (1962).

Many researchers are also seeking answers to the narcolepsy problem by studying the reticular formation (Moruzzi and Magoun, 1949; Hobson, 1974). The reticular formation is a complex structure of nerve cells running from the spinal cord to the brain stem to the brain. This formation or network serves two major functions: activation and inhibition. One system encourages the onset of sleep while the other tends to prevent sleep. Researchers are proposing that lesions or changes in this structure, such as injury to the brain stem, may predispose a person to narcolepsy or, in fact, may cause a full-blown narcoleptic disorder. An injury of this sort generally can cause disturbances of consciousness. Narcolepsy is certainly a disturbance of consciousness: for example, narcoleptic sleep attacks and hypnagogic hallucinations constitute major changes of consciousness, while cataplexy and sleep paralysis are narcoleptic phenomena in which the nature of one's consciousness is affected by unusual conditions.

The state of knowledge about precise anatomical locations of brain lesions in narcolepsy is, at present, hypothetical. Yet it is generally agreed upon that the problems of the reticular formation play an important role both in narcolepsy proper and in the NREM-REM, or non-dream to dream cycle of sleep. In narcolepsy, sleep is disordered and normal dream cycles are disordered as well. These functions of the brain are largely regulated by the various activating and inhibitory functions of the reticular formation. For example, the Ascending Reticular Activating System (ARAS) regulates different levels of the awake states from drowsy to altogether alert. In order for sleep to occur, the ARAS must be functioning at a low enough level so that the sleep system may be activated.

Narcolepsy itself, has not been treated by direct surgical intervention on the brain or direct treatment of any injury to the reticular formation. Its only treatment other than psychotherapy is with medication. (The use of drugs in narcolepsy will be discussed in Chapter 8.)

Bonstedt (1954), who also recognizes that narcolepsy research is in its infancy, suggests location sites in the brain that may cause narcoleptic problems. He relates functions of the diencephalon portion of the brain to the functions of the reticular formation and suggests how this relation may produce narcoleptic symptoms. The diencephalon contains autonomic nerve centers that regulate involuntary responses such as those of the involuntary muscles. Bonstedt believes that a full biophysiological and anatomical understanding of narcolepsy will be possible only when the entire physiology and function of sleep are better understood.

Dement (1972), in analyzing the narcoleptic syndrome, has suggested that *all* narcoleptics also have cataplexy but that the motoric inhibition and the behavioral and subjective aspects of the REM-dream sleep attacks "are so well synchronized that cataplexy or sleep paralysis never occurs separately." What this means is that sleep paralysis may actually be a variation of cataplexy itself, insofar as in both there exists a muscular paralysis. Thus, those narcoleptics who do not experience cataplexy per se, but do experience sleep-paralysis, may, in fact, be having cataplectic attacks that appear in the form of sleep paralysis. It should be remembered that in both cataplexy and sleep-paralysis consciousness is maintained but one's voluntary musculature is temporarily paralyzed.

Dement suggests that cataplexy and sleep paralysis are really dissociative manifestations of the motor inhibition process. This means that consciousness is separated from the process that temporarily paralyzes the muscles. This motor inhibitory process is a normal part of sleep so that cataplexy and sleep-paralysis must contain, in their underlying physiological structure, some important mechanisms of sleep. In this same vein, several researchers have shown that cataplexy, sleep-paralysis and hypnagogic hallucinations occur during REM-dream sleep and that cataplexy shows the same rapid eye movements seen in narcoleptic sleep. Apparently, the rapid eye movement feature of dream sleep may accompany each of the narcoleptic symptoms. Dement's proposal implies, therefore, that in narcolepsy there are times when one is physically asleep and mentally awake simultaneously. Dement (1965, 1972) also discusses the biological role of rapid eye movement sleep, and Brock and Wiesel (1941), in an early study, correlate symptoms of narcolepsy with dissociated reactions of the sleep mechanism.

The hypnagogic hallucination is also considered to be a dissociative or split-off feature of motor inhibition. As a matter of fact, the hypnagogic hallucination is considered by many sleep researchers actually to be a dream. The specific relationship of hypnagogic hallucinations to dreams as well as nightmares will be considered in the following chapter.

The hypnagogic hallucination may also reflect some component of so-called *D* sleep or deep sleep, which occurs during motoric or muscular inhibition in the absence of all other biophysical features of sleeping. This means that the hypnagogic hallucination may be a dream that the narcoleptic has while mentally awake but physically asleep. This manner of understanding hypnagogic hallucinations contains important diagnostic implications for the meaning of narcolepsy. These implications will be discussed in the section on narcolepsy and schizophrenia, also presented in the following chapter.

The foregoing discussion has attempted to show that a physical basis for the appearance of narcolepsy is being widely considered. Furthermore, scientists are also beginning to search for various brain function locations that, when interfered with, can cause the narcoleptic disorder. In the following section, the psychogenic or non-physical theories of the development of narcolepsy will be described.

A PSYCHOLOGICAL BASIS FOR NARCOLEPSY

Psychological or psychogenic narcolepsy is called *idiopathic* (Mitchell, Dement and Gulevich, 1966). Idiopathic literally means not caused by any other disease. In the case of the narcoleptic disorder it means not caused by any physical or organic damage. Many authors have suggested that various life *transition* themes can cause narcolepsy:

for example, leaving home for the first time, first sexual experiences, dissociative reactions, strong dependency feelings, career changes, graduation from school, and marriage have been cited as possible causes for the appearance of narcolepsy. More specifically, authors have attributed this disorder to Freudian or psychoanalytic themes. For example, persons who have been attacked but who are fearful of retaliating may repress their rage and frustrations. When feelings such as rage are repressed, they then can form into a symptom—in this case a narcoleptic symptom. Another psychoanalytic theme of the relationship between narcolepsy and personality refers to the issue of family attachments—the kind analysts call *symbiotic*. The symbiotic relationship refers to the overdependence of family members on one another. *This kind of dependent-symbiotic relationship is so exaggerated that narcoleptic symptoms may develop when family members are separated.* The narcoleptic symptoms therefore, would be an expression of *separation anxiety*.

Authors have written papers with respect to the emotional components and neurotic nature of narcolepsy (Morgenstern, 1965; Missriegler, 1941). Some have even proposed that a narcoleptic syndrome may appear in people who have an abnormal fear of death—which also refers to the extreme form of separation fears. Other psychoanalytic themes attributed as causes of narcolepsy have been fear of homosexuality, a wish to kill, and a wish to rape—extreme causative elements, to say the least. Further, Barker (1948) has discussed narcolepsy with respect to the personality dimensions of dependence versus independence; Levin (1953) has attributed the narcoleptic attack to an "attack wish"; Sours (1963) relates narcolepsy to passive-aggressive features and flat affect; Vogel (1960) discusses the REM attack as an expression of fantasy gratification; and Palmer, in an early study (1941), correlates narcolepsy and hysteria.

Morgenstern (1965) considers narcolepsy to be an excellent example of a psychosomatic disorder, a point also proposed by Smith (1958). This means that narcolepsy ultimately generates physical incapacities but in essence is caused by psychological and emotional tension. Orthello, Langworthy and Betz (1944) also refer to narcolepsy as a response to severe emotional conflicts.

In the latter part of the 19th century, Charcot and Freud analyzed narcolepsy with respect to sexuality. Examples of the nature of sexual impulses attributed to narcoleptic persons may be compiled from psychoanalytic writings on this subject.

> One such description is of a 48-year-old woman whose narcolepsy was attributed to an incestuous experience in which she reports that her father and she had intercourse during her adolescence. This woman started having repetitive dreams of coitus with orgasm. Another case in the scientific literature is of a person with sleep hallucinations consisting of the feeling of being masturbated. A third case cites a narcoleptic person who, during each daily nap, would experience a seminal emission. This person was essentially having a sexual wet dream. Still a fourth case describes a man who would experience erection at each sleep attack. Finally, psychoanalysts interested in the effects of symbiotic relationships on psychosomatic disturbances cite cases in which the patient would fall asleep whenever discussion of the patient's mother was started. One such case occurred in the psychoanalyst-patient relationship: the patient became dependent on the analyst and would fall asleep instantly if the analyst suggested that they discuss this dependency.

Other cases of treatment with psychotherapy, descriptions of psychodynamic aspects of narcolepsy, and even proposed psychodynamic aspects of disturbances in the sleep mechanisms are offered in Coodley (1948), Davison (1945), and Farber (1962). Among psychodynamic theories, incest or sexual impulse themes are examples cited as psychological causes of narcolepsy but they are by no means universally accepted.

Sigmund Freud, in his analysis entitled *Dostoevsky and Parricide,* (1927) even suggests that sleep attacks may be incited by unconscious murderous wishes in those people who are hysterical personality types. By hysterical types Freud presumably means people who are easily influenced, who tend to deny feeling angry, and who can develop many psychosomatic disorders. The analysis by Freud suggests that sleep itself is a symbol both for death of the parent and for self-death. The wish for one's own death serves as a punishment for dreadful death wishes against the parent. Thus, to Freud, narcolepsy is a perfect solution for this sort of conflict. The narcoleptic sleep becomes a symbol of one's personal death as a retribution and punishment for harboring bad wishes toward one's parents.

Another feature of the psychological symbolism of narcolepsy refers to the meaning of humor as understood from a psychoanalytic framework. Morgenstern (1965) points out how Freud related unconscious motives in humor to anger or to sexuality. Freud suggested that hostile wit represented aggression and obscene wit symbolized sexual exhibition. This relation between aggression and humor has been affirmed by most psychoanalytic writers since Freud. Many narcoleptic patients express hostile wit. Furthermore, narcoleptic patients are likely to repress their anger; when they do, a narcoleptic symptom is quite likely to appear in its place. Thus, a psychological basis for the appearance of sleep attacks has been attributed to dependency, separation, sexual and anger effects.

The psychological basis for sleep-paralysis and hypnagogic hallucinations was related to dreams and nightmares by Jones (1949). Jones believed that the hypnagogic hallucination, in fact, was a nightmare.

THE RELATION OF HYPNAGOGIC HALLUCINATIONS AND NIGHTMARES

Liddon (1967) indicates that a comparison of the present day understanding of attacks of sleep-paralysis and hypnagogic hallucinations with older descriptions of nightmares "leaves little doubt that sleep paralysis and hypnagogic hallucinations were important features of the nightmare." Freud, in *The Interpretation of Dreams* (1900), called the nightmare and its associated inhibited motor (or muscular) condition a "conflict of will." Jones further suggested that Freud really implied an inherent connection between the feeling of dread and repressed sexual impulses, and he defined the nightmare as a condition reflecting maximum repression. What this means is that Freud's implicit theory of narcolepsy (or sleep attacks) and its relation to sexual incestuous impulses is carried forth into the nightmare in the form of the feeling of dread. Freud proposed that strong sexual impulses would be defended against by turning them into opposite feelings. Thus, revulsion and dread can actually imply a sexual feeling that was turned into its opposite. A person experiences dread and revulsion because of presumed real feelings of a sexual nature which, because of their incestuous flavor, are unacceptable. Because of such unacceptability, Jones defined the nightmare as a dream that reflects maximum conflict. He suggested that the experience of motoric and muscular paralysis accompanying the nightmare, as well as the sleep paralysis of the narcoleptic, represented a person's defense against or avoidance of such sexual and incestuous wishes.

In the psychoanalytic literature, motoric inhibition is considered to be a defense against or an avoidance of masturbation. The fear of masturbation becomes a fear of incestuous fantasies. Thus, the sleep-paralysis presumably successfully accomplishes the avoidance of masturbatory inclinations.

Of all the biological as well as psychological theories of narcolepsy, the most convincing seems to be the position that narcolepsy is caused organically but that it is also significantly affected by personality and life stresses.

Narcolepsy is a disorder that psychologically can be controlled to some extent through psychotherapy and can also be chemically managed through drug therapy. Thus, narcolepsy seems to be a biologically based disorder with a very definite psychological and emotional overlay. Those physicians and therapists who recognize the reciprocal interplay of both these forces will be in a better position to treat this disorder.

A PSYCHOSOMATIC SYNTHESIS OF NARCOLEPSY

In an early study Davison (1945) conducted laboratory investigations of sleep disturbances, and concluded that no matter what sort of repressed unacceptable wishes exist in the narcoleptic person, they can precipitate the narcoleptic disorder only if they create prolonged emotional anxiety. This anxiety will result in the appearance of nervous system symptoms such as sleep disturbances, of which narcolepsy is a prime example. Morgenstern (1965) and Smith (1958) also suggest the psychosomatic connection in narcolepsy.

> ". . . narcolepsy is centered about unacceptable impulses and defenses they provoke. In cataplexy episodes, sexual and aggressive actions and fantasies are blocked on a neuro-muscular level. A sleep attack is far more complicated and some aspects may be compared to a classical psychoneurosis because the symptom provides not only defense but simultaneous disguised gratification of a wish" (Morgenstern, 1965).

It is proposed here that narcolepsy appears to be a disorder rooted in physiological anomalies and either aggravated or minimized by the extent to which psychological and emotional factors play a part in its appearance. The diagnostic implications of this disorder, the use of drugs in the treatment of narcolepsy, and a case illustration of the psychosomatic, or perhaps better, the somato-psychic nature of this disorder, will be presented in the following chapter.

Chapter 6

Psychiatric Diagnoses Related to Narcolepsy: A Case Illustration

NARCOLEPSY AND PSYCHIATRIC DIAGNOSES

Psychotherapists treating narcoleptic patients have generally applied only a few basic diagnoses to these patients. One such diagnosis considers the narcoleptic to be a person suffering from considerable tension and anxiety and one who has a number of physical complaints. This high level of tension and anxiety will eventually be expressed through symptoms such as those of narcolepsy.

Those persons who express such tension experience psychologically and emotionally based symptoms such as loss of consciousness, paralyzed limbs, swallowing problems, and a host of other so-called *conversion reactions*. These reactions do just that—they convert anxiety and tension into bodily symptoms, so that an underlying conversion structure may be attributed to the narcoleptic's personality.

Another diagnosis applied to narcoleptic patients relates to the presence of unusual fears; for example, Morgenstern (1965) pointed out that a narcoleptic patient he had seen was extremely afraid of dogs, deep water, and birds, and he made the diagnosis of *phobic reaction*. What this means is that the patient's anxieties were transformed into abnormal fears. In this case, the fear or phobia may be considered to be somewhat related to the conversion reactions. Both the phobic and the conversion reactions can also be aspects of what may be called the *hysterical personality*.

Another basic diagnostic description attributed to the narcoleptic patient's personality refers to the frequent observation that such patients are sometimes stubborn individuals who tend to oppose the influence of other people. They may also exhibit sarcastic and caustic traits and show a tendency to be highly critical towards others. This means that a narcoleptic patient with this sort of personality structure tends toward being angry and hypercritical. This type of personality involving these specific features is generally defined as *paranoid-like*—that is, someone who is intractable, stubborn and critical. As has already been outlined, narcoleptic persons who are dependent and passive are frequently unable to express dissatisfactions directly so that large amounts of anger accumulate and this anger is slowly and indirectly released. Sarcasm, stubbornness and oppositionalism are examples of derived traits stemming from the poor management of anger.

> Paul, the narcoleptic patient previously discussed, was evaluated with the Rorschach inkblot test. Results showed that he was a rather guarded and suspicious person whose store of anger and oppositional attitudes was so strong that he could have easily lived by the motto "reject first before you're rejected." The responses he offered to the inkblots further showed that he was somewhat withdrawn and depressed and although he was a very sentimental person, his overall emotionality seemed severely restricted. His personality strongly reflected a critical style that was expressed throughout the test.

The remaining diagnostic characteristic of narcoleptic individuals in whom dependency, passivity, and aspects of inadequacy or immaturity are central is that of *depression*. The aspect of depression in narcoleptic persons is an underinvestigated element of diagnosis. The dependent personality has been described in earlier parts of this book. This is the kind of person who has become accustomed to relying on parental support and who may also be exceedingly passive. In addition, the *inadequate personality type* may be someone who has a high intelligence but who underresponds in virtually every aspect of life. In this sense, the inadequate personality type is associated with a person who has not developed to full maturity in life and who usually fails at tasks, does poorly in social situations, and shows great occupational incapacity with respect to the achievement of any personal aims. These characteristics may also apply to narcoleptic persons with severe dependency problems.

Although it is not a universally accepted premise that all narcoleptic individuals share the same underlying personality structure, nevertheless many narcoleptic patients seem to show depressive elements in their personalities and many are subject to overeating and to gaining weight. Most times this increased appetite and subsequent weight gain are due to the side effects of medication. However, it is not clear whether increased weight is solely due to medication. It should also be noted that dependency needs, weight gain as a result of eating problems and the diagnosis of depression constitute one major unit or syndrome in psychoanalytic conceptions of personality. As far as overeating is concerned, Morgenstern (1965) even reports that the only time his patient could count on staying awake was while eating.

In the following section, a case of narcolepsy in a man of 40 whose diagnosis basically reflects mixed features of the above mentioned diagnoses will be presented. The patient is a critical type who also displays symptoms of anxiety. In addition, he is socially immature and tends to respond inadequately in numerous situations. He is profoundly unable to do what he sets out to do and occasionally displays deeply ingrained depressive elements in his behavior.

A CASE HISTORY OF A NARCOLEPTIC PATIENT

Conditions Leading to Narcolepsy

Ralph entered treatment at the age of 26, referred by his family physician. He was experiencing bouts of depression and exhibiting what seemed to be classic, full-blown narcoleptic symptoms.

His depressive feelings had emerged about one week after he had rented his own apartment for the first time. It was the very first occasion that he was on his own except for the time he spent in the Army several years before. As it turned out, he did indeed have a history of drowsiness dating back to high school, but had never experienced any true narcoleptic symptoms. His decision to leave home seemed to have caused his depressive feelings. At the time, this *separation* was the only notable event immediately preceding the onset of his narcoleptic symptoms.

Ralph's narcolepsy probably did not first emerge when he left home for the Army some years before because in certain important respects the military became a substitute *care* station for him. He was really not separate and on his own: There were regulations to follow, authorities who were responsible for him, and a sense of mutual support with other recruits. When he left home to live in his own apartment, an entirely different set of conditions were created. There was no surrogate mother or care-station available and he was entirely on his own; there were no regulations to follow, no one was responsible for him, and, there was no sense of community or mutual support from other people who were in the same "trench." He was actually alone. All in all, given Ralph's particular personality configuration, the new separation conditions were just right for the onset of narcolepsy.

Family and Social History

Ralph was raised in a mid-western city. His family was an upstanding community-minded one. Ralph was a middle child, with an older brother and a younger sister. Ralph's sister was born when he was five and it was then that Ralph felt his "life was over." He was a terribly dependent child "right from the beginning" and remembered feeling excluded from the bosom of the family starting at about the time his sister was born.

During his elementary school days, whenever his schoolmates played together, he would tag along but sensed that he also wanted to be home with his mother. In reminiscing, Ralph concluded that of all the people he had ever known, he felt himself to be the most dependent. During adolescence when his friends started dating, he was embarrassed to talk to girls. When he managed to galvanize himself to ask someone for a date, he would literally begin by saying, "You wouldn't want to go out with me Saturday night, would you?" This attitude indicated that Ralph's inferiority feelings were already quite developed at adolescence. In general, Ralph's adolescent years were occupied with watching television each weekend. He never really dated but was preoccupied for many years with fantasizing and masturbating.

His relationship with various family members was cordial although physical affection in the form of hugging and kissing—even as greeting or parting gestures—was absent. His father, a merchant seaman, was away from home most of the time. His older brother, who was also a loner of sorts, nevertheless managed always to find a girlfriend. His sister was also able to form adequate relationships.

All three siblings were generally lazy about schoolwork. They were bright, but quite passive and undersupervised with respect to homework and other responsibilities. As a result Ralph was a mediocre C student. He attended college with the same result. Yet, he was quite literate and his natural writing ability was usually recognized by his teachers in both high school and college. His main problem was that he could not get himself to begin his writing assignments or to submit material on time.

The Onset of Narcoleptic Symptoms

Within one week of leaving home, Ralph became depressed. Within one month he noticed on several occasions that he would experience "an overwhelming pressure to sleep." One day while having lunch in a restaurant and reading a newspaper, he could not help but overhear a bickering argument between a husband and wife at the next table. When the wife offered her husband a very sarcastic but salient rejoinder to one of his parries, Ralph experienced his first cataplectic attack. One night shortly thereafter, while preparing for bed, he turned off his lamp and began to go to sleep when he suddenly, and for no apparent reason, seemed possessed by a total sleep-paralysis. He also immediately experienced a hypnagogic hallucination in which he hallucinated his employer entering his apartment and "standing at the door gazing." Ralph tried to say, "What are you doing here?" but he could not move or speak. The next day at work Ralph felt quite awkward talking to this man because he was not quite sure whether the previous night's experience was a dream or whether it had really happened. In the course of the year, Ralph also experienced sleepwalking as well as fugue episodes with automatic behavior. He also had occasional insomnia at night when he should have been sleeping. Thus, Ralph showed a full classic narcoleptic picture.

His psychological and emotional conflicts centered around overabundant dependency feelings, great loneliness, and a profound inertia. He was an overeater and tended to gain weight. He used his intelligence in the service of a razor-sharp wit which, when excercised, would trigger cataplectic attacks in himself. He was singularly unable to tell anyone directly how he felt about them. He kept things in and he brooded. He could never put his exceptional talent for writing to good use because he felt severely inadequate, dependent and restricted. He was always concerned that what he wrote was never quite good enough or did not express what he intended. This exaggerated self-doubt simply reflected his inability to view himself as an independent person who could initiate activity on his own. Rather, he saw himself as a little boy who had never really grown up. He depended on his mother to do things for him and felt secure only when he was around her.

His mother was initially the one who suggested he rent an apartment because he was never dating and she felt he would remain unmarried. He moved to New York and obtained employment as a television market-researcher. His job was to monitor one TV program after the other while sitting in a darkened studio in order to see if brand names of commercial items were mentioned on programs which were not sponsored by those brands.

It was an interesting job at first, but after a while the monotony of sitting in a darkened room generated a whole host of narcoleptic sleep attacks. He was accused of sleeping on the job and fired because his list of unsponsored commercial slips was consistently smaller than the average amount on the comparable lists of other such employees.

During a therapy session, Ralph commented, "the irony of it all—they got me for sleeping but for the wrong reason." The punch line prompted a cataplectic attack—he fell back in his chair and lost control of his muscle and motor ability. The attack lasted about 20 seconds after which time he gradually recovered. All the while, his eyes were closed and his lids exhibited the rapid eye movement typical of narcoleptic and cataplectic attacks as well as the rapid eye movement exhibited during dreams.

Adolescent-Incestuous Sexual Experience

During the first year in treatment Ralph was most preoccupied with complaining about those circumstances in his life that made it difficult for him to become successful. He was unwilling to acknowledge that his self-defeating sarcastic style would have to be modified in order to minimize his cataplexy. He was also unwilling to see that he would have to become more forthright with his feelings if he were to expect any progress in minimizing his narcoleptic sleep attacks.

Ralph was mostly a blamer. Yet, there was an integrity about him that was appealing. It was this honesty that ultimately permitted him to view his situation with greater perspective and to hold in abeyance excessive critical feelings he was having toward people. During such times he could think about his problems and seemed more mature. He usually denied feeling particularly anxious and did not really admit to feeling anything intensely at all. His denial of feeling intense emotions was also true when he talked about masturbation. In his masturbatory activity, he would from time to time engage in a single fantasy, but he nevertheless claimed that most of the time he masturbated in an automatic fashion without thinking of any fantasy. He did, however, occasionally describe what he considered to be the most exciting sexual event in his life—the only one he has remembered when masturbating.

Apparently, starting at the age of 10, whenever his aunt, his mother's sister, would visit, she would room with him and they would share his bed. At that time she was approximately 30. She was a single woman, who, he said was beautiful. She would ask him to massage her legs, which, she claimed, ached. Ralph would spend what he felt to be hour upon hour just sitting next to her in bed rubbing her legs. He freely admitted feeling intensely sexually excited by this and he never complained that it was taking too long. He reported that she would ask him to do it "all the way up—higher," and that it was not uncommon for him to inadvertently end up touching her vagina while ostensibly rubbing her thighs. He remembers that sometimes she would lie on her stomach and at other times on her back. His most exciting memory of these incidents involved getting close to her upper thighs and beginning to touch her pubic hair. She would occasionally moan or she would say that it felt good. Ralph would simply and slowly continue massaging her. He claimed nothing more ever happened. The massaging incidents lasted until he was 14 at which time she married and moved away.

During these sexually awakening adolescent years, Ralph's contact with his aunt provided him with the only pleasurable and exciting memories of his childhood. He never told his mother about them and to this day he believes no one ever knew what was happening. Ralph is still not sure whether his aunt ever felt his hands on and around her vagina. He also still maintains that she was an innocent woman who needed rubs for her aching legs while he was the one with the hidden sexual agenda. He felt he was gratifying himself with someone who truly did not realize what was happening. During those years he would masturbate compulsively while thinking about his aunt. It is still his only masturbatory fantasy.

The Freudian dynamics of this repeated experience in Ralph's life concerns the sexual impulses released in him toward a family member—one who could easily be a mother replacement. As mentioned in an earlier section of this book, sexual impulses—especially incestuous ones—are thought by some psychoanalysts to be the cause of the narcoleptic's psychological conflicts. Yet, it is highly doubtful that all or even most narcoleptic persons actually have had such incestuous experiences. Thus, the psychological meaning of incestuous experiences as they relate to narcolepsy may be only one of many that apply to the psychodynamics of narcolepsy.

Other than the intense sexual feelings Ralph described about his aunt, his emotionality during therapy sessions was always moderate. He seemed to be sedentary, a bit withdrawn and depressed. Oddly enough he would describe himself as a friendly and sociable person even though he was actually quite isolated.

In order to better understand the discrepancy between how he actually appeared and how he saw himself, Ralph consented to undergo a series of psychological tests. Some were administered by a psychologist at a sleep clinic, some by a private consulting psychologist, and some by Ralph's therapist. In the following section the pertinent findings of these tests will be presented.

Psychological Test Results

A comprehensive battery of tests was administered in order to gather information with respect to three major issues. First, the nature of Ralph's emotional integration was examined—that is, whether he was able to respond with appropriate emotion, whether he could express a typical range of emotions, and whether his emotion had depth. Second, the basic configuration of his diagnosis—especially with respect to depression and hysterical and paranoid tendencies—was drawn. Finally, tests were administered to determine whether Ralph's narcolepsy had a conventional organic basis; such tests show whether responses given by persons with organic physical deficits correspond to the test responses Ralph offered.

Tests Administered

Personality tests to evaluate the nature of Ralph's emotionality and diagnosis included:

(1) *The Rorschach Test*. This test, known as the inkblot test, is a procedure in which patients are asked to describe the impressions inkblots remind them of. Through a highly specialized analysis of what, where, and why certain perceptions were seen, a comprehensive picture of personality patterns can be developed.

(2) *The Thematic Apperception Test*. In this test, patients are presented with pictures that depict a scene, usually involving people doing something. Patients are asked to create a story using each scene as a basis. Information regarding personality features, attitudes, needs, and defensive mechanisms—that is, the coping strategies that the patient uses—may be derived from the analysis of the stories.

(3) *The Figure Drawing Test*. This test requires the test-taker to draw the figure of a person. Artistic skill is not what is important here. A great deal about one's personality may be revealed from this test both with regard to diagnosis and the test-taker's means of adjustment in day-to-day living.

(4) *The Minnesota Multiphasic Personality Inventory*. This is a short-answer test in which patients are asked to recognize statements that may apply to their particular preferences and behavior in life. This test offers information on the extent to which the test-taker expresses attitudes and needs of a variety of basic diagnostic categories.

(5) *The McAndrew Scale*. This test is also a diagnostic one. Responses to this test offer the possibility of comparing the test-taker to other special problematic clinical groups.

(6) *The Beck Depression Inventory*. This test is used to determine the patient's level of depression and the nature of the depression.

(7) *The Emotions Profile Index*. This test can determine the extent of one's emotional restriction and the level of conflict between specific opposite emotions. It can yield information with respect to depression as well as other basic diagnostic categories. Subjects choose personality adjectives that best apply to them. Through a special scoring technique, an *emotion picture* is developed of the test-taker.

(8) *Baron's Ego-Strength Scale*. This test measures a person's ability to cope with stress. It can yield information specifically designed to guage the emotional maturity of the test-taker.

(9) *The Bender Gestalt Test*. This test requires the subject to copy geometric figures. There is a sufficient amount of background material on this test to enable an individual's results to be compared to the results derived from patients with physical or organic brain deficits, brain damage, or lesions, whether they are minimal or great.

(10) *The Owl and Lark Questionnaire*. This test is tailored to determine the sleep cycle inclinations of the test-taker. It reveals whether the subject is basically a morning type or an evening type.

Thus, of the 10 tests administered to Ralph, some were designed to derive overall personality information, others to examine his emotionality and diagnosis, while still others to determine whether his narcolepsy was correlated to any apparent physical dysfunction.

Diagnostic Considerations

Ralph's diagnostic picture is not a simple one. It contains many features, the most striking of which, even more than his very significant depressive pattern, is the state of his withdrawal. The Rorschach test revealed a profound element of withdrawal in him, together with a strong repressive need. Thus, his tendency, as mentioned previously, is to avoid managing or coping with situations in a mature, direct manner. Results on the Rorschach supported this hypothesis and even suggested that the sleep symptom of narcolepsy works very well in reinforcing his withdrawal and repression; he sleeps instead of confronting tensions more directly and maturely. In this sense, his narcolepsy is not necessarily the cause of his withdrawal; rather, it services the withdrawal by making it easier to carry out. This type of withdrawal is usually caused by severe or traumatic events early in a person's life. The birth of Ralph's sister when he was five years old and his inordinately negative overreaction to this event could conceivably qualify as one such traumatic event. His extreme feeling of abandonment at that time also implies that his relationship with his mother must have been highly tenuous for it to be so easily and devastatingly threatened by his sister's birth. Ralph's solution to this conflict was, and remains to this day, his isolated and guarded attitude.

Furthermore, the Rorschach shows Ralph's responses to be essentially critical and they reveal him to be a dissatisfied person. His high measure of criticality implies that he also feels guarded and these qualities are part of a paranoid approach. The Rorschach also suggests that his guarded feelings are expressed through his depression and in his feelings of agitation. In other words, he is depressed, in part, because he is dissatisfied, and this constant dissatisfaction generates the agitated condition. He expresses agitation and criticality by being stubborn, oppositional, and unable to accept advice easily.

On the Emotions Profile Index (Plutchik and Kellerman, 1974) an experiment was designed with Ralph. He first took the test by responding to test items in terms of the way he felt they actually applied to him. This produced an emotions profile that was highly restricted with respect to his capacity to experience pleasure and to be sociable.

In Figure 6.1A the pleasure restriction is seen in his Self Emotions Profile insofar as his Gegariousness and Trustfulness scores are significantly lower than normal. In contrast, he perceived himself to be somewhat depressed, critical, stubborn or paranoid, and this corresponds to how he saw himself in the Beck Depression Inventory. His Emotions scores of Depressed, Distrustful and Aggressive are all significantly higher than normal.

He was then asked to retake the test, this time as though he were imagining himself to be the kind of person he would want to be ideally —in other words, in terms of his ideal-self. Results of this part of the experiment revealed a higher and perfectly normal pleasure score and a decrease of the negative emotions (Figure 6.1B). Apparently, even though Ralph can imagine how it would be to feel happier, less critical, and less restricted, he nevertheless cannot, in reality, be like that. The interesting and important finding here was that Ralph indicated he could tell he was not what he wanted to be. This indicated that he indeed had some insight into his "emotional-appearance."

The third part of the experiment was one in which the therapist took the Emotions Profile Index test for Ralph; that is, the therapist based his responses to the test items on how he personally perceived Ralph with respect to Ralph's natural and characteristic everyday behavior. The results were astonishing. The picture of Ralph on the basis of these results was of someone depressed, highly angry, critical, guarded, and profoundly restricted in all positive and social emotions. This result is reflected in Figure 6.1C in which the pleasure scores are almost completely restricted while his depression obviously dominates his emotional picture.

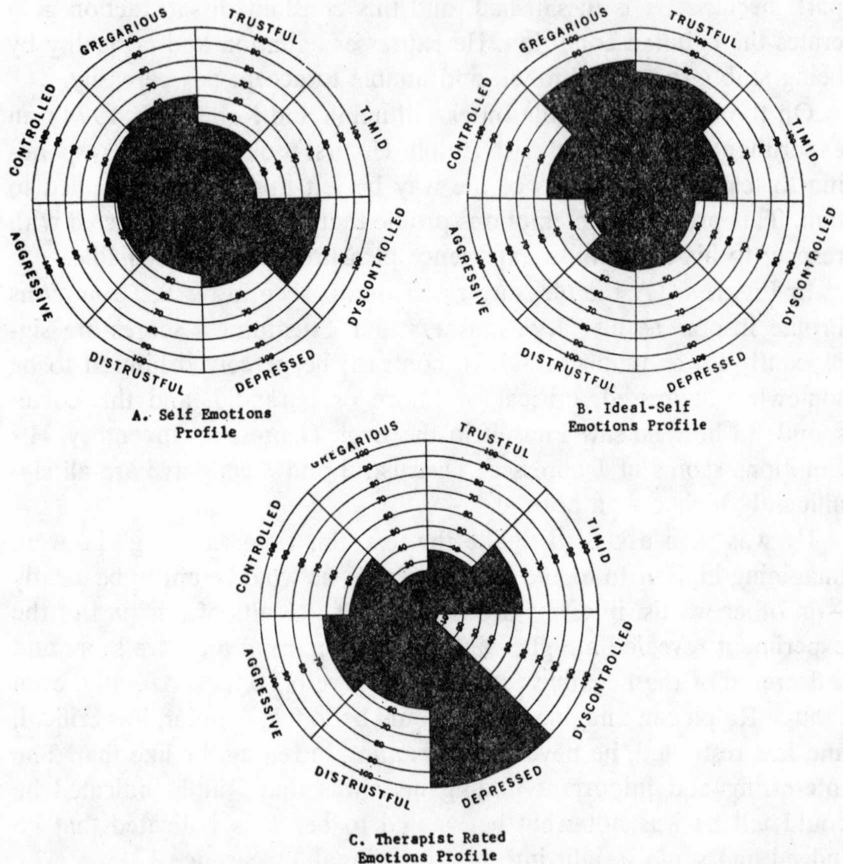

FIGURE 6.1: Emotion profiles showing a profound discrepancy between patient's self-perception and the therapist's perception of him—especially with respect to the variable of depression. The center of the circle represents zero percent and the outer ring of the circle represents 100 percent.

It became clear that Ralph's pervasive withdrawal, emotional constriction and depression were only somewhat visible to him; that is, he was severely depressed and withdrawn but unable to fully appreciate his dilemma. His symptoms of narcolepsy certainly could have been reinforced by this personality configuration. The question to be asked from this experiment becomes: How is it possible for someone to be so severely withdrawn and depressed and not to really see it? The answer to this question is revealed in the results of most of the tests.

The Key to Ralph's Inability to Perceive His Severe Depression

First of all, the Thematic Apperception Test shows that only superficial feelings are attributed by Ralph to any character of the stories. Whatever feelings are ascribed to individual characters are shallow; emotion is present only because of the logic of the story. Second, results on the Minnesota Multiphasic Personality Inventory revealed the existence of a pathological depression. Yet, test results showed that Ralph refused to acknowledge any faults in himself, even common, minor flaws. This suggests that he feels vindicated in his beliefs and in his critical behavior. He apparently needs to feel justified in his criticism of others and his assertion of his own pureness of intent. His stubborness therefore, is masked (as suggested by one of the testers) in an "uncompromising moral stance." In other words, he justifies and rationalizes all his dissatisfactions by blaming others. In everyday behavior this problem is expressed in an attitude of condescension and through a style of sarcasm. He readily accomplishes his aims of blaming, and the Baron's Ego-Strength test indicates that he possesses ample coping abilities. Yet, he is dependent. On various tests such as the McAndrew Scale he emerges with dependent personality features resembling those characteristic of drug addicts or alcoholics. On the one hand, through his condescension and sarcasm he behaves imperiously and on the other he feels like a vulnerable needy child.

Third, he is unable to see his depression, also because he lacks significant emotional interaction in his life—he is socially isolated and thus somehat *schizoid*. He is somehat anhedonic—that is, restricted in terms of pleasure. He is quite successful in his display of emotional control and this explains his higher ego-strength coping score on the Baron's Ego-Strength Test. Yet the single most important feature of his personality—the one that accounts for his inability to view his own depression—is his self-absorption in the form of withdrawal, reinforced by the poor integration of emotionality in his personality.

What this means is that Ralph cannot, in a healthy way, manage emotional reactions, so he controls them, holds them in abeyance, represses them, and ultimately develops psychosomatic symptoms about them. His narcolepsy is complicated, therefore, by an arbitrary integration of emotionality. The net effect of such emotional isolation is that eventually this sort of withholding or denial of emotions can generate physical symptoms.

The emotional short circuit between Ralph and the rest of the world can be defined as one in which he may feel emotion, but goes about hiding it, transforming it, being arbitrary about it or repressing it. He may, in fact, at first feel the emotion, but he quickly transforms it, so that what others see is only what is left: a stoic, unemotional, withdrawn-schizoid and depressed person.

The Hysterical Feature of Ralph's Personality

On some of the tests, Ralph's intellectual ability, or I.Q., may be estimated by the number and quality of his responses. Beyond any doubt, Ralph has a high I.Q. On an intellectual level he can generate many responses and some very interesting ones at that. Part of this high production of responses is a result of his underlying store of energy. The Figure Drawing test showed this in interesting ways. His figures were well controlled but they contained features that implied a spilling over of impulses not unlike the figure drawing impulse signs typically offered by patients whose impulses do tend to find a kind of action outlet, such as epileptics. His figures were immature and showed features of extreme dependency and inordinate need for control. They revealed that despite his critical stance toward the world he is basically quite frightened and potentially susceptible to suggestion and external influences. The one sign on the Figure Drawing test suggesting any organic condition was this impulse-spilling-over sign.

Signs of Organic or Physical Damage

The Bender Gestalt test as well as the Figure Drawings—all the graphic tests that are frequently used to diagnose brain damage—did not reveal any hard-core signs of brain deficit or damage. There were present, however, so-called soft-signs of some physical problem, and even the one diagnostic indicator mentioned to suggest the possibility of a subtle impulse-spilling-over organic disorder. His particular disorder of narcolepsy, however, could not be seen as a bona fide brain injury problem from these tests. The Owl and Lark test showed him to be an extreme morning type. Results on this test, however, by implication, perhaps point to some problem in his sleep-dream cycle. His *circadian cycle*—or internal body clock—is thus upset to an abnormal extent. He frequently sleeps when he should be awake. This sense of regulation and "programmed" time is discussed also by Conroy and Mills (1971) in terms of circadian rhythms, and by Luce (1971) who calls it "body time." A 24-hour rhythm is also identified in a study of depression (Phlug and Tolle, 1971) and the entire subject of biological "clocks" is treated by Richter (1965). Other references to circadian rhythms are presented in Chapter 12 in a discussion of good sleep versus bad sleep.

In this clinical test illustration of Ralph's personality organization, a picture emerges of a person in the grip of a painful dilemma. He desperately wants to be cared for, yet isolates himself. He thinks that people will see him as friendly and sociable, yet he is powerfully depressed and isolated. He would like more social interaction, but defeats this aim by acting condescending, sarcastic and stubborn. He is very bright and would like to be accomplished, yet he can't help falling asleep on his job. One of the more difficult problems he has is wanting to raise a family, but a side effect of the medication he is taking to control his narcoleptic symptoms is a partial impotence. Unfortunately, the problem of selecting proper medication is a difficult one, in part because of occasional deleterious side effects that can impair one's sexual potency.

In summary, one can see the debilitating and demoralizing effect of narcolepsy. It can threaten one's job, relationships, and any chance to lead a normal family life. Some authors even claim that it can threaten one's grip on reality and lead to a breakdown. In the following chapter, the possible relationship of narcolepsy to schizophrenia is discussed. In addition, the relation of the hypnotic process to narcolepsy is presented and how these comparisons may reveal the deeper diagnostic meanings of this disorder is suggested.

Chapter 7

Schizophrenia and Hypnosis: Their Relation to Narcolepsy

SCHIZOPHRENIA AND NARCOLEPSY

It is true that sometimes narcoleptic individuals may also be schizophrenic—but this possible association with schizophrenia can also apply to diabetics, cardiac patients, and people with any number of other disorders. Yet some authors have theorized that narcolepsy is actually an equivalent form of schizophrenia—that narcolepsy develops instead of schizophrenia (Farber, 1962; Smith, 1958). This proposed substitution process of narcolepsy for schizophrenia prompts the phrase *schizophrenic-equivalent,* or one disorder for another. The idea is highly speculative and is based upon the similarity of some narcoleptic symptoms to schizophrenic ones (Brock and Wiesel, 1941).

Schizophrenia is a condition known as a thinking disorder. In schizophrenia, one may experience changes in consciousness, delusions and hallucinations; in one form of schizophrenia, even one's voluntary muscles are affected. These changes in thinking and in physical phenomena are all symptoms also seen in narcolepsy. In narcolepsy, one's consciousness is frequently affected, especially as a result of sleep-attacks. In addition, consciousness changes such as hallucinations of the hypnagogic variety emerge during the sleep-paralysis attack. These hallucinations are so vivid that they are mistaken for real events. Although not quite as extensive as a delusion, nevertheless this mistaken belief certainly contains delusional-like qualities (McKellar and Simpson, 1954; Schacter, 1976; Slight, 1924; Vihvelin, 1948).

In catatonic schizophrenia, an individual may become frozen in one position—paralyzed as it were—unable to move at all. This problem of muscle paralysis or muscle inhibition resembles the paralysis seen in cataplexy or in the narcoleptic sleep-paralysis attack itself. Because of such behavioral symptom similarities, several cases have been cited in the psychological literature that propose the substitution theory between narcolepsy and schizophrenia. Interestingly enough, in those cases that draw this connection, it is only the narcoleptic syndrome that is considered to be an aspect of the schizophrenia, while the schizophrenia is considered to be the substitute disorder. The diagnosis usually attributed to this kind of schizophrenia-substitute narcolepsy is of the paranoid variety.

> Farber (1962) cites a case of a male patient in his early 40s who exhibited most of the classic narcoleptic symptoms except hypnagogic hallucinations. This patient is reported to have had a long-standing, intensely close relationship with his mother and to have shared a bedroom with her. He became highly withdrawn and isolated and was depressed most of the time.
>
> The diagnosis of schizophrenic reaction with narcolepsy was based upon his condition of narcolepsy in conjunction with the appearance of various schizophrenic signs. The patient suffered from schizophrenic illness characterized by thinking disturbances, severe emotional disturbance, great indecision, and withdrawal from reality, accompanied by an increase in his fantasy life. His narcolepsy and cataplexy were considered also to be symptoms of his schizophrenia. Most of his attacks occurred after encounters with aggressive women.

The above clinical description of this man, simply interpreted, means that he became governed in his behavior more by his fantasy, daydreams, or imagination rather than by everyday reality. His deep depression constitutes a severe emotional disturbance. His indecision means that he was never really able to be independent or assertive; rather, he would be equivocating and apprehensive, and would become exceedingly tense whenever he felt he had to meet the expectations of others. This is generally referred to as "ambivalence." Ascribing his cataplectic attacks to encounters with aggressive women is perhaps an oblique reference to his dependent relationship upon his mother and the repressed anger implied by this dependency. Thus, his cataplectic response to women he perceives as dominant may really be a submissive display—falling at the feet of another person—that only symbolically contains the expression of anger and corresponding penance. Another way of understanding this is to suggest that the cataplectic attack is an attempt to achieve forgiveness for bad thoughts and bad feelings. Of course, his symbolic response to women who are characterized as being dominant is consistent with passive, submissive, and anger conflicts that can be attributed to narcoleptic persons of this type. As described in previous chapters, this sort of person is frequently reported to have had extreme mother attachments with unconscious incestuous feelings, and to be excessively critical. There is sometimes a paranoid quality to these feelings—that is, a constellation of traits that go together, including criticality, hostility and guardedness. Such a constellation of conflict leads to the proposition that such people are deeply angry but do not know it and, therefore, cannot directly manage it.

As a matter of interest, Smith (1958) notes that all psychoses or mental illness associated with narcolepsy are of the paranoid schizophrenic type with narcolepsy appearing prior to the psychosis. Smith, as well as Sours (1963), also indicates that the narcoleptic person is frequently an extremely passive person. Other sleep researchers and therapists who have treated narcoleptic patients would most likely agree to the correspondence of passivity and narcolepsy. In certain respects the trait of passivity in the narcoleptic person is to be expected, especially since cataplexy can always be set off by some excitement. The narcoleptic's need for "quietude" may create conditions that encourage the development of passive as well as dependent features of personality.

Yet, there is a basic difference between a narcoleptic person and a person with schizophrenia, even though in certain respects symptoms of both appear to be alike. Although some authors conceive of the narcoleptic state as part of a schizophrenic disorder, nevertheless it should be emphatically stated that narcolepsy per se may be as different from schizophrenia as cataplexy is from epilepsy. Yet, other studies such as those by Drake (1949), Eilenberg and Woods (1962) and Zarcone (1973) generally indicate that attempts to differentiate narcolepsy from schizophrenia are essentially inconclusive. However, there is one major and fundamental difference between narcolepsy and schizophrenia which will be presented in the following section.

A Basic Difference Between Narcolepsy and Schizophrenia

Freud points out in *The Interpretation of Dreams* (1900) that a person must be asleep in order to dream. The dream disregards the logic of time—past, present or future—and it disregards the logic of age and place. In the dream you can walk on water, become aged, become the opposite sex, and even be yourself while simultaneously also appearing as another person. You can be married to some unlikely figure and, even with the realization of the absurdity of these roles and circumstances, nevertheless the dream proceeds with its peculiar story line, symbols and terrors, or whatever preposterous events that are occurring. All of this is permissible because, as is universally known, anything can happen in a dream. Since one is asleep, then such abnormal events do not count. The occurrence of these absurd events in dreams does not mean that one is crazy or schizophrenic or even in any way abnormal. Yet, what would happen if one were dreaming while awake? Such a person would be talking illogically, or perhaps running from some dangerous pursuer whom no one else is able to see. Such conversations and actions would be real to the person experiencing them, while to an onlooker they would seem like signs of craziness. Such conversations in thin air, however, do in fact occur in the awake state, but not with narcoleptics. They occur in the awake auditory and visual hallucinations of people suffering from a schizophrenic disorder—frequently of the paranoid variety. And this asleep-awake dichotomy in the appearance of such symptoms is the basic and fundamental behavioral and physiological difference between schizophrenia and narcolepsy.

A schizophrenic person may have a dream in the form of an hallucination *while awake*. The narcoleptic person who also experiences an hallucination—and a vivid hypnagogic one at that—remains sleeping, in a state of partial sleep, or, at least in a state of reduced consciousness. So long as one dreams while asleep or under the hypnotic influence of sleep, then one is quite normal. The products of the dream as it emerges in the schizophrenic patient can occur while the patient is awake. As such, it is a full-blown hallucination. Many people have at some time observed another person having what is called an hallucinatory episode, walking in the street and in a somewhat bizarre way conducting an animated, even rageful, conversation with the air. Actually such a person is having an auditory hallucination. When questioned during more tranquil moments, such persons are likely to report that, in fact, they actually heard someone speaking to them and they were quite naturally answering. At other times, persons with angry fantasies toward others may feel them so intensely that during stressful moments they lose sight of where they are and begin to *talk-out* their hostilities toward these people instead of simply thinking about them. This sort of experience can occur in anyone. However, the actual talking to and hearing of "messages" is a different and abnormal experience—a schizophrenic one.

As can be seen, the narcoleptic person is suffering from a different sort of disorder. The irrationalities that all individuals experience and express in dreams while asleep remain for the narcoleptic just that—irrationalities of dreaming while asleep or while in a paralytic sleep-like state. For the schizophrenic person who hallucinates, such irrationalities burst through into consciousness while awake, causing such persons, in fact, to be diagnosed as schizophrenic and *not* narcoleptic. The narcoleptic person, therefore, should not be considered schizophrenic solely on the basis of symptom similarities. Were narcoleptics to experience dreams while awake in the absence of compelling needs to sleep, or in the absence of the sleep paralysis condition, then such individuals would not be narcoleptic, would be having bona fide wide-awake hallucinations and then could be considered as possibly schizophrenic. In the narcoleptic person, dreams are greatly overproduced; therefore, such persons are dragged into sleep—as in the narcoleptic sleep attack—*in order to dream.* If such people did not sleep, they may hallucinate. The point is, however, that they do sleep while dreaming.

NARCOLEPSY AND HYPNOSIS

Narcolepsy also resembles the hypnotic state; that is, certain classic features of narcolepsy are also found in the process of hypnosis or in the process of *going under*. This narcolepsy-hypnosis relation is an obvious connection to make because the process of hypnosis in some ways resembles *a going to sleep and yet being awake state.*

The induction of hypnosis resembles the expression of a narcoleptic condition in several ways. The person undergoing hypnosis is somewhat like a narcoleptic person whose symptoms can be controlled. The entire process of *going under* in hypnotic trances may be roughly divided into six stages (Sarbin, 1972; Wolberg, 1948). Each of these stages produces effects that resemble some aspects of narcoleptic symptoms.

The first stage in the hypnotic process is a *drowsiness stage*. Here, a person undergoing hypnosis begins to experience a lethargy and a comfortable relaxation. At this first stage, what is known as catalepsy of the eyes takes place. Catalepsy is similar to cataplexy, but in catalepsy a single limb or organ of the body can remain in one position; for example, subjects can be instructed to close their eyes and keep them closed, and generally that subject's eyes will remain closed. In this first stage of the hypnotic trance or sleep, eye catalepsy will occur.

In the second stage of the trance, the subject will be in a *light sleep,* somewhat deeper than during the first stage. During this second stage, arm catalepsy can be observed. If a subject is asked to lift a limb such as an arm and keep it in a particular position, the instruction or suggestion will usually be followed and the subject's arm will remain fixed in this position until that subject is instructed to change position.

In the third stage the subject will be essentially *asleep,* although able to hear and respond to the hypnotist. This sleep will resemble normal sleep.

In the fourth stage, the subject will be instructed to go deeper into sleep and will, in fact, go into a *deep sleep.*

The fifth stage is one in which the subject can sleepwalk. This stage may be called a *somnambulism* one. During this stage, a subject can be instructed to experience what is known as a positive hallucination—that is, the subject can be asked to see a clock on the wall when, in fact, no clock exists.

The sixth stage may be called a *profound somnambulism stage* in which the subject can be asked to obliterate the perception of a clock on the wall when a clock actually does exist. This last stage may be called a *negative hallucination stage*—not seeing something that is, in fact, actually there.

These hypnotic trance stages are similar in many ways to aspects, symptoms, or processes of narcolepsy; for example, the drowsiness of the hypnotic first stage resembles the drowsiness preceding narcoleptic sleep-attacks. The arm and eye catalepsy of the hypnotic stages one and two resemble the muscular anesthetization appearing during sleep-paralysis and during cataplexy. The sleep of hypnotic stages three and four resembles the state of hypnagogic hallucination appearing during sleep-paralysis because during these deeper stages hypnagogic states can be produced.

All in all, there are essentially four criteria for judging the depth of the hypnotic trance, and most of these factors are also diagnostic features of the narcoleptic disorder. These criteria of judging the hypnotic trance depth are: (1) the presence of catalepsy; (2) the capacity to produce an amnesia for events; (3) anesthesia with respect to pain, and, (4) the capacity to produce hallucinations. A sequence of tests is used to judge the depth of any trance (Gill and Brenman, 1959). These include: (1) eye catalepsy or keeping the eyes in one position (this focus on eyes is similar to the importance given to rapid eye movements in testing for the appearance of dreams during the narcoleptic sleep-attack); (2) arm catalepsy, or the yielding of control of the musculature of the arm to given instructions (this yielding of control over muscles of any limb resembles the loss of control of musculature observed during cataplectic attacks); (3) amnesia for name or number that resembles the forgetting of dreams during sleep-paralysis and narcoleptic sleep-attacks, along with automatic behavior, in which amnesia for events and behavior characterize the symptom; (4) analgesia of arm or hand which resembles the sleep paralysis symptom—the limb in this case is literally asleep; and, (5) both positive and negative hallucinations which, of course, correspond to the narcoleptic hypnagogic hallucination.

These comparisons between the hypnotic trance and the narcoleptic syndrome are in some cases more compelling and in other cases somewhat more speculative. The main point, however, is that the comparison between both states may suggest some additional insights into narcolepsy. For example, with respect to the physiological implications of the state of consciousness, it is interesting to note the studies that have been made on the carotid sinus and its relation to the basis of consciousness (Moller and Ostenfeld, 1949). The carotid artery on the side of the neck can prevent blood from reaching the brain; if sufficient pressure is applied to this area, a subject will lose consciousness. It is an anatomical location that may also be used as a pressure point in hypnosis to facilitate the hypnotic trance. Furthermore, it has been reported that narcoleptic patients exhibit twitching and tic-like behavior directly around the shoulders and the carotid sinus area. Narcolepsy, the hypnotic process and the function of the carotid sinus —all in some way either affect consciousness or are states in which the effects of altered expressions of consciousness are seen.

SOME DIAGNOSTIC VARIATIONS OF NARCOLEPTIC PERSONS

The relation between hypnosis and narcolepsy may reveal additional insights into the basic nature of narcolepsy. One question raised by this comparison refers to the adaptational quality of narcolepsy; that is, can narcolepsy actually help a person? The narcoleptic sleep symptom acts as a release mechanism, giving the narcoleptic sufferer a chance to withdraw and perhaps thereby to cope with tensions. Actually, this is not a farfetched idea. There are some theories of schizophrenia that propose a similar formulation—that a breakdown can help a person escape from unmanageable tensions. In this sense, schizophrenia is considered to be a protective coping solution to anxiety. Thus, according to some theorists, schizophrenia and other diagnostic states are actually considered to be helpful coping devices or are considered to be adaptational. These disorders become coping compromises between the experience of tension and the relief of tension.

Although there is really no massive or convincing evidence to support this theory, it nevertheless raises an important question with respect to the underlying purpose of any disorder. For example, in physical illness, the purpose of a fever is not just as a signal of infection. A fever galvanizes the functions of the body—the body metabolizes at a faster rate, rids itself of wastes faster, uses up nutrients faster—all in the service of fighting the infection. The fever is a symptom both of the infection and of a bodily coping mechanism or temporary adaptation to the infection. Similarly, the narcoleptic disorder can also be considered as a signal of some more fundamental conflict. It, too, may be both a symptom as well as a mechanism designed to cope with some more basic problem. For example, the similarity between narcolepsy and the stages of the hypnotic trance suggests that somewhere within the underlying personality structure of persons with narcolepsy may lie what can be called an hysteric element. It is the suggestibility feature of personality that facilitates the hypnotic trance in persons diagnosed as hysterical types: the more suggestible one is, the more easily one is hypnotized. This further implies that not everyone can be hypnotized because some people are quite stubborn, controlled, and intractable—far from being suggestible. The more one is rigid, stubborn and critical, the less is the possibility of being hypnotized. In contrast, the less one is rigid, stubborn or critical, the better is the chance of being hypnotized.

The one diagnostic type that is highly suggestible is the hysteric type. On the other hand, the one diagnostic type that is least suggestible is the paranoid type. These two diagnostic types—the hysteric and the paranoid—are opposites. The interesting point about these diagnostic types is the paradox they reflect when they exist in one person. More simply, the following question can be asked: Since most features of the hypnotic trance resemble those of the narcoleptic condition, then why are hypnotic types more often diagnosed as hysteric while persons with narcolepsy—especially depressed, passive and dependent types—more often diagnosed as paranoid? How can the process of hypnosis and the disorder of narcolepsy in depressed or passive dependent persons be highly similar in symptoms and features when the basic nature of their respective diagnoses is quite opposite? The answer may be that the diagnosis of persons who can be hypnotized and the diagnosis applied to such narcoleptic persons are only *apparently* different.

It may be that beneath the paranoid, critical and stubborn facade of the narcoleptic person who is depressed and dependent there exists a highly suggestible personality. Interestingly enough, dependency features of personality contain elements of both suggestibility and criticality. Thus, dependent features of personality can viably exist in the hysteric as well as in the paranoid. This implies that a narcoleptic person who is a dependent type but who may show paranoid-like traits of criticality and stubbornness can on some deeper level harbor features of an hysterical disposition—that is, of someone who may really be suggestible. The correlation between narcolepsy and hysteria is also discussed by Palmer (1941).

If this simultaneous existence of paranoid and hysteric features is so, then the psychological defensive purpose of narcolepsy may be revealed. Here, *defensive* is defined as a coping or protective use of a personality trait. It may be that such a narcoleptic person has a great fear of allowing deeply underlying suggestibility features to surface. This means that such a person may need to protect or defend against the emergence of a true hysterical personality pattern. This emergence is defended or protected against because it could cause such a person to feel vulnerable to surrounding events. It could even evoke a fear of injury. Because of strong dependency needs, one can feel vulnerable to social demands so that a paranoid or guarded defense perimeter is constructed at one level of the personality. This is done in order to reduce the possibility of both seeming to be and becoming vulnerable. The paranoid-like pattern of sarcasm, criticality, and stubbornness is one that obviously creates a shield or field around a person so that any *suggestion* or possible influence from the environment will have little if any effect. A person's vulnerability is, therefore, well protected.

According to this interpretation, a narcoleptic person is revealed to be one who does not seem to be subject to influence. This narcoleptic paranoid personality structure protects such a person from extreme vulnerability to any suggestion and influence from others. The interesting phenomenon about narcolepsy itself, however, is that virtually any narcoleptic person can be hypnotized instantly This supports the proposition that the narcoleptic individual no matter how stubborn on the surface—is highly suggestible underneath. As a matter of fact, the narcolepsy syndrome itself is one that favors monotony and sleep—factors which also facilitate the hypnotic process. Thus, the narcolepsy and the paranoid personality in which it is occasionally wrapped may be fundamentally a transparent attempt to guard against feelings of suggestibility and hysterical vulnerability.

These speculations about the various personality features of narcolepsy and the possible coping nature of this structure indicate that the range of narcoleptic personality features is complex and perhaps not easily treated. Such complexity also makes for great difficulty in the prescribing of medication. Is medication prescribed for underlying depression, for anxiety, for the alleviation of the sleep attack problems, for the control of cataplexy, for possible schizophrenia, or for a combination of these? Will one kind of medication be successful for one narcoleptic symptom but aggravate another? Are there any untoward side effects of the medication prescribed for the narcoleptic problem? Some of these issues shall be considered in the following chapter.

Chapter 8

The Use of Medication in the Treatment of Narcolepsy

There are several drugs that have been used to treat the psychological and emotional problems of narcoleptic patients as well as the specific symptoms of the narcoleptic tetrad. It seems that the most common treatment decision with narcolepsy is primarily to address its physical symptoms. Treating the emotional problems of narcoleptic patients is usually a secondary consideration. It is helpful, therefore, to be familiar with the pharmacology of problematic sleep to better understand the pharmacology of narcolepsy (Kay et al., 1976; King, 1971; Oswald, 1968; Zung, 1970).

The drugs used to treat narcolepsy are usually chosen to control the narcoleptic sleep attack and to decrease the frequency of cataplectic attacks (Hishikawa, Eida, Nakai and Kaneko, 1966; Kales and Kales, 1974; Karacan, Moore and Williams, 1979; Yoss and Daly, 1959). There are essentially four such drugs that have been used most frequently in the treatment of this disorder. Each of these has had various degrees of success and can also, interestingly enough, be prescribed for persons who are depressed and withdrawn (Physican's desk reference, 1978). A further description of the issue of medication and disordered sleep is presented in Chapter 14, and a greater detailed analyis of dosage prescription and side effects of medications is given in the Physician's Desk Reference as well as in Honigfeld (1973), Klerman and Paykel (1970), and Rech and Moore (1971). An analysis of the use of tricyclics in narcolepsy is also offered in Cadilhac (1976) and Takahashi (1976).

TYPICAL DRUG TREATMENT FOR NARCOLEPSY

Elavil

Elavil or *amitriptyline hydrochloride* is one such antidepressant tricyclic drug. It is effective with chronically depressed persons. It also has been used to treat narcolepsy and in some cases it is reported to have completely eliminated the attacks of cataplexy as well. One of the troublesome side effects in the use of Elavil is that in some patients there will be a tendency for increased appetite, thereby producing weight gain. The usual amount prescribed is a 25 milligram dose three times a day for a total of 75 milligrams. Weight gain from 15 pounds to about 30 pounds or more has been reported.

> Mark, diagnosed as a narcoleptic, was originally prescribed Elavil by his family physician on a slightly higher dosage than recommended. His narcolepsy practically vanished but he became extremely agitated; he could not stop talking and moving around. He developed a lot more twitching to his already exhibited narcoleptic twitching and he became unusually restless. The major problem, however, was high weight gain. He was a well-built man on the stout side to begin with. At six feet tall, he weighed 195 pounds. After several months on Elavil, he had gained 65 pounds. When medication was discontinued, he began to reduce immediately, but his narcolepsy and cataplexy both returned with an unusual ferocity and he had many more attacks both of sleep and cataplexy.

Elavil, then, although quite effective for the relief of physical symptoms of the narcoleptic disorder, can produce adverse effects in emotional intensity and in increased appetite. Even when the dosage is adjusted, these effects are still observed, although to a lesser degree. The effect of Elavil on narcoleptic symptoms also reveals an interesting aspect of narcoleptic sleep attacks. When sleep attacks are suppressed, then the REM (rapid eye movement) dream attacks are also suppressed. Any drug that will halt the sleep attacks will also be stopping the overabundant narcoleptic onset of REM. The phenomenon that has been observed with respect to this REM suppression, however, is that when patients cease ingesting REM suppressant drugs they then have what is called *REM rebound* (Mendelson, Gillin and Wyatt, 1977). REM rebound is the appearance of many more REM periods than usual. These seem to replace or make up for those REM periods that have been lost; for example, in a six- to eight-hour night of sleep, the number of REM dream periods is likely to double. Instead of four or five dream periods, there are likely to be eight to ten. This rebound occurs after treatment with the antidepressant drugs and the monoamine-oxidase inhibitors (MAO), as well as with the tricyclics which suppress or entirely eliminate REM. The MAO's are the most powerful suppressors of REM.

Tofranil

Tofranil, or *imipramine,* is another tricyclic anti-depressant drug designed to relieve depression. It is found to lessen the frequency of cataplectic attacks. The problem with Tofranil is that occasionally it too may cause a hyper-energized, agitated or manic tendency. If the dosage is too high, it can also cause insomnia, numbness, and tingling sensations. Tofranil has been used to control cataplexy effectively, but there is no general agreement about its effectiveness in the treatment and control of narcoleptic sleep attacks. It also may have negative side effects insofar as increased appetite and consequent weight gain can create problems. The typical dosage in the use of Tofranil is 25 milligrams three times per day for a total of 75 milligrams.

Dexedrine

Dexedrine, or *dextro-amphetamine,* is one of the most frequently used medications for narcolepsy. However, it usually does not help reduce the number of cataplectic attacks. Dexedrine may be habit-forming for some people and it may cause withdrawal symptoms. It is not recommended for those who are agitated and it may in some cases generate side effects of insomnia and restlessness. Yet, it is partially effective in the treatment of narcolepsy and it is often presented in dosages of 5-10 milligrams to be taken three or four times per day.

Ritalin

Ritalin, or *methylphenidate hydrochloride,* is also an energizer and psychostimulant. It is used for mild depressions, lethargy and withdrawal, and is reasonably successful both with narcolepsy and cataplexy. It is not recommended for persons with intense anxiety or for those who are agitated. Ritalin is also not recommended for persons with severe depression, and it, too, can be habit-forming. It can produce insomnia, general nervousness and muscle twitching. Dosages are given twice or three times per day for a total of up to 100 milligrams. It is recommended that the last dose of the day be taken early enough so that it does not interfere with regular night sleep.

SIDE EFFECTS OF MEDICATION AND OTHER TREATMENT CONSIDERATIONS

Table 8.1 presents a summary of clinical data on a variety of patients with narcolepsy who were on a regimen of amphetamines (Roberts, 1970). This table also shows other associated clinical symptoms. In a recent study, Parkes (1976) has presented an analysis of the relation between amphetamines, alertness and narcolepsy.

> At one time or another Mark has taken each of these drugs in addition to several others such as Esquatril and Dexamile. He has experienced most or all of the side effects described above. The most effective drug treatment for Mark has been a combination of Dexedrine and Ritalin. He is now taking 10 milligrams

TABLE 8.1

Summary Of Clinical Data On 12 Patients With Narcolepsy Who Ingested Excessive Amphetamines

AGE	SEX	OCCUPATION	AMPHETAMINE DOSAGE (DAILY)	DURATION OF NARCOLEPSY	CATAPLEXY	SLEEP PARALYSIS	HYPNAGOGIC HALLUCINATIONS	FAMILY HISTORY OF NARCOLEPSY	HYPOGLYCEMIA	CAFE-AU-LAIT SPOTS	OTHER CLINICAL FEATURES	RESPONSE TO RX
21	M	Student	45 mg	4 years	+	+	+		+	+	Reading disability; driver impairment; psychiatric features	Good
27	M	Upholsterer	"Addicted"	9 years	+		+		+		Driver impairment; obesity; diabetic G.T.T.	Good
45	F	Registered Nurse	30 mg. +	5 years			+	+	+		Recurrent edema; diabetic G.T.T.	Good
31	F	Housewife	40 mg. +	14 years	+	+	+	+	+	+	Alcohol intolerance; recurrent edema; cerebral dysrhythmia; diabetic G.T.T.	Good
28	F	Teacher	50 mg. +	4 years	+		+	+	+		Unnecessary thyroid; previous obesity; driver impairment; recurrent edema; psychiatric features; cerebral dysrhythmia; diabetic G.T.T.	Good
36	F	Housewife	50 mg. +	5 years	+	+	+		+	+	Recurrent edema; phychiatric features; previous alcoholism; cerebral dysrhythmia; diabetic G.T.T.	Required psychiatric institutional care
27	M	Engineer	30 mg. +	10 years	+	+	+		+	+	Obesity	Good
22	M	Student	45 mg. +	"All my life"	+	+	+		+		Psychiatric features; diabetic G.T.T.	Good
39	M	Salesman	50 mg. +	20 years	+	+	+	+	+		Obesity; previous alcoholism; diabetic G.T.T.	Good
43	F	Housewife	60 mg. +	"All my life"	+	+	+		+	+	Recurrent edema; psychiatric features; previous obesity	Good
32	M	Physician	Up to 100 mg.	10 years	+	+	+		+		Needless thyroid; alcoholism	Refused treatment
36	M	Minister	30 mg. +	10 years					+	+	Diabetic G.T.T.; dumping syndrome (partial gastrectomy)	Good

Adapted from: Roberts, H. J. Unrecognized narcolepsy and amphetamine abuse. *Medical Counterpoint*, August 1970, 28-42.

> of Dexedrine per day as well as 20 to 40 milligrams of Ritalin per day. His narcoleptic symptoms are still experienced, but to a lesser extent. Despite his regular program of medication, when Mark feels that job requirements make extraordinary demands on him, his anxiety rises and his narcoleptic sleep attacks increase. When he feels only minimal demands, his symptoms are in turn minimized.

Another significant side effect of the various drugs taken for narcolepsy is the effect they have on sexual activity.

> After taking Elavil for some time, Mark reported difficulty in maintaining an erection and a sudden inability to ejaculate even when he could maintain an erection. He also experienced an overall decrease in his sexual inclinations—a decrease of libido. This effect was alleviated after the cessation of this drug, but his sexual functioning was not fully restored until some time had passed.

Medication for nacolepsy is only partially successful. If the narcoleptic person is also diagnosed as schizophrenic, then Ritalin and Dexedrine do not seem to be effective. In such cases, the use of Thorazine or *chlorpromazine* seems to address both the schizophrenia as well as the narcolepsy. Thorazine frequently stabilizes persons diagnosed as schizophrenic in the absence of narcolepsy. Those schizophrenic persons with narcolepsy may also be helped by Thorazine because of the REM-dream inhibiting effect of this drug; the suppression of REM-dreaming activity will then inhibit the need for sleep if there is no inordinate need to dream. Although Dexedrine and Ritalin also suppress REM-dream activity, they do not simultaneously address the biochemical involvement in schizophrenia.

Finally, and most encouragingly. Broughton and Mamelak (1976) have indicated that use of Gamma-Hydroxy-Butyrate has led to a reduction of the narcoleptic sleep attack, cataplexy, hypnagogic hallucinations, and sleep paralysis—the entire narcoleptic tetrad. This substance is non-toxic and metabolizes within three or four hours. The claim is made that Gamma-Hydroxy-Butyrate normalizes the etntire sleep cycle in the beginning stages of the night and thus recalibrates the patient's circadian rhythm. It is thought that because it duplicates REM periods at night and essentially generates a coherent nocturnal sleep pattern, the entire narcoleptic symtom tetrad will subside during daytime hours—a suggestion that narcolepsy may be a nocturnal sleep problem at its foundation.

Another interesting aspect of narcolepsy theory concerns the diet of the narcoleptic. It has been suggested that narcolepsy is really caused by hypoglycemia. The theory proposes that fatigue, lots of coffee, and an excess of water and alcohol should be scrupulously avoided by narcoleptics. Corrective measures that have been suggested include eliminating sugar from one's diet and assuring that the narcoleptic should not be without food for more than three hours—day and night (Roberts, 1970).

All of the theories advanced to determine a treatment regimen for narcoleptic patients are tentative. A general consensus about how to treat narcolepsy is just beginning to form. This consensus is based upon the correct use of medication along with a beginning awareness of the usefulness of psychotherapeutic support.

AN INCOMPLETE SLEEP DIARY

The extreme difficulty experienced by a narcoleptic patient in exercising single-minded determination in the pursuit of any goal or in cooperating with the treatment for this disorder is illustrated by the following *sleep diary* Mark tried to keep for several days. As it turned out, he could not stick to the task and what developed was a partial and inadequate sleep record over several days. Mark wanted to keep this record for purposes of deciding how to best regulate his medication. This record would include his intake of medication, hours of nighttime sleep, narcoleptic sleep attacks and cataplectic attacks during his daytime activities, attacks of sleep-paralysis and the appearance of hypnagogic hallucinations and other narcoleptic sleep variations that may have occurred. As it turned out, Mark found it most difficult to keep a complete record. He responded in the way he usually responded to assignments—with motivation and good intentions that soon became tinged with resentment and an inability to implement or complete the assignment thoroughly. His first attempt at recordkeeping produced a two-day record that was drastically incomplete.

10/23—20 mg. Ritalin 9:30 A.M.
20 mg. Ritalin 10:30 A.M.
Light drowsy on way to restaurant in car 2:30.
11:37 P.M. went into sleep-paralysis while getting ready to sleep for the night. Came on very quickly. Dreamt very soon at the end of paralysis and at the end of regular sleep. Don't remember any [dreams].
10/24—20 mg. Ritalin 9:00 A.M.
10 mg. Dexedrine 4:00 P.M.
Light sleep in subway 4:30-5:00.

Mark's first attempt at diary-keeping was obviously incomplete and demonstrated his difficulty in sticking to a task. The first day's record failed to indicate one cataplectic attack which he described during the therapy session. He also mentioned that he had three or four narcoleptic attacks between 2:30 in the afternoon and the time he went to sleep for the night. As a matter of fact, that entire period of time from 2:30 until his bedtime is omitted in the diary.

Mark indicated he wanted to try keeping a diary once more since he realized that his difficulty in keeping records was an example of the same problem he was having with everything else he tried to do. He simply underresponded to practically every activity in his life—especially with respect to work demands. Mark's next attempt to keep a diary was more complete and it demonstrated his seriousness of purpose. It was a hopeful sign of his potential ability to respond to what he considered work pressure. He was extremely happy that he could maintain his focus on the diary for one full week even though he felt that the second attempt still fell short of his goal.

11/29—40 mg. Ritalin 7:00 A.M.
Slight drowsiness 1:00 P.M.
4:00 P.M. Damn near a full-fledged attack. Very

sleepy. Just about made it to men's room to sleep (about 5 mintues). Still quite groggy upon return to desk. Fell asleep after about 5 minutes on subway. Awoke approximately 30 minutes later. Still intermittent sleep for 10-20 seconds.

6:30 took a nap because I felt tired. I had only about three hours sleep Tuesday night. (Mark has bouts of insomnia whenever he has had many sleep-attacks during the day). Woke up at 8:00 P.M. Back to sleep for night at 10:30.

11/30—20 mg. Ritalin 7:00 A.M.
10 mg. Dexedrine 12:00.
Middle drowsiness at noon. Shook it off and took a Dexedrine. Felt good getting on subway. Slept a bit but not too much. Slept from 7:20 to 8:10. Had "heavy teeth" dream.

12/1—20 mg. Ritalin 7:00 A.M.
10 mg. Dexedrine 12:00.
Generally good all day. No heat at home. Got into bed early to keep warm. Slept from 9:00 to 9:40.

12/2—Woke up about 10:00. Took a Ritalin. Mostly stayed in bed to keep warm. Made love from 12 to 1. Slept from 4:00 to 5:00—fairly deep sleep. Was extremely tired at 11:00 P.M. Slept until 2:00 A.M. Up for an hour.

12/3—Ritalin—11:00. Not too tired all day. Took bus home. Had cataplexy on bus. A lady was cursing out some man who wouldn't give her a seat. He told her to "get lost" and I then had the attack. Got home O.K. No pressure (meaning no compelling need to sleep) but slept approximately one half hour.

12/4—1 Ritalin 7:00 A.M.
1 Dexedrine 12:30
Generally speaking not too tired all day. Stayed at work until 7:30. Not tired. Slept lightly for 20 minutes on bus going home. The noon pill is generally necessary during workdays only.

12/5—2 Ritalin 7:00 and 3:00 P.M. Had pressure at 5:30. Slept deeply 15 minutes.

This diary is an example of the kind of problems some narcoleptic patients have in maintaining an equilibrium between their periods of sleep and periods when they are awake. Mark's medication regimen was working very well for him. His cataplectic attacks were well controlled. His therapy work succeeded in limiting a strongly developed condescending attitude that in the past would frequently trigger cataplectic attacks. His increased assertiveness also helped him to gain a measure of control over his problem. It is hoped that this mini-diary illustration will convey some flavor of the daily difficulties faced by narcoleptic persons.

Narcolepsy can be partially controlled by medication and, to some extent, also by psychotherapy. At this point, however, there is no known cure for it. Yet there is such a ferment in sleep research and research into sleep-related problems that narcolepsy may in the near future, be cured completely. As noted above, one of the most recent developments in this treatment is the report of Broughton and Mamelak (1976) on the use of Gamma-Hydroxy-Butyrate which is reported to have had a profound ameliorative effect on all the symptoms of narcolepsy. One of the problems narcoleptic persons face, however, is the difficulty many physicians have in diagnosing this disorder. As previously mentioned, it is frequently misdiagnosed as lethargy, anxiety, depression and neurasthenia.

At present, the most impressive improvement in the condition of narcolepsy results from a combination of medication administered with careful attention to side effects along with psychotherapeutic treatment. It is important that the physician and psychotherapist be experienced in the treatment of this problem. It is hoped that this book will provide a broad introduction to the narcoleptic disorder so that physicians and psychotherapists may be able to recognize it more readily and treat it more effectively.

Part III

INSOMNIA

Chapter 9

Insomnia: The Staying Awake Problem

"I JUST CAN'T SLEEP!"

There are no uniform statistics agreed upon by sleep researchers regarding the number or percent of insomniacs in this country. Some estimates place the number of true insomniacs at about 30 million or about 15 percent of the population. These are presumably people who are severely troubled by their inability to feel rested after a night's sleep. Yet if all those who are tortured sleepers were added to those who are poor sleepers, restless sleepers, and sleepers who awaken earlier than they expect to, closer to 50 million people or more would be included (Bixler, 1976; Luce and Segal, 1969; Ware, 1979). Insomnia and related problems can be considered epidemic in their proportions (Kales et al., 1974; Karacan and Williams, 1971).

Statistics regarding sleeping (Baekeland and Hartmann, 1970; Karacan et al., 1976; Webb, 1970) suggest that the average person sleeps seven and one-half hours per night. Five to 15 percent of the population—about 10-30 million people—sleep fewer than six hours per night, while the same number sleep more than nine hours. Many people who complain of sleeplessness usually sleep less than six hours per night. Some of those who sleep more than nine hours also complain of poor sleeping and consider themselves to be insomniacs who spend all of that sleeping time in search of a true good night's sleep (Kales et al., 1972; Ware, 1979).

The insomniac's lament of "I just can't sleep" is a catchall phrase for an entire spectrum of stay-awake problems. There are many kinds of insomniacs and many ways to classify them. Some truly do not get enough sleep and some, in fact, do sleep, but do not feel refreshed upon awakening (Hauri, 1970). The latter see themselves just as troubled about their sleep as those who actually cannot get to sleep in the first place. Sleep is a very personal matter and someone who is troubled by sleep problems does not want to be told that it is an imaginary problem or that it does not compare in importance to the more severe sleep problems that others have.

No matter what kind of insomnia one experiences in a subjective sense, people who cannot sleep would like to slow-up the night so that they may still have a chance to get some good sleep before the night passes. Even those who dread the night and pray for daylight in order to end their ordeal would, in a more primary sense, want to retard the progress of the night in the hope of eventually sleeping. The true insomniac is tortured by this problem, tosses and turns in bed, may watch the clock throughout the night, and usually dreads the prospect of bedtime.

The insomnia attributed to children at holiday time, vacation time, or special event times such as birthdays is only euphemistically referred to as insomnia. Children experience the excitement and expectation of the following day during such times and their loss of slumber is short-lived. At times, this kind of temporary sleep disorder of children may even be counted in minutes, an hour or two, or an evening at the most. Under such circumstances, the primary wish in the child is to speed up the night. Children hardly ever worry about not getting enough sleep. Thus, children's so-called insomnia is not usually authentic insomnia. The true insomnia of the adult who watches the clock minute for minute and who, sooner or later, hears all the things that go bump in the night is the real subject of this discussion. In the following section, various kinds and types of insomnia will be described.

TYPES OF INSOMNIA

The problems of insomnia are roughly divided into three broad categories (Luce and Segal, 1969). These are: (1) problems of falling asleep; (2) problems of staying asleep; and, (3) problems of early awakenings. The classic insomniac, of course, is known as the first type who cannot get to sleep and who will swear that each minute of the night was consciously experienced. The second type occasionally complains of not being able to get to sleep. The major focus of the complaint, however, is that after sleeping for awhile, an awakening takes place in the middle of the night in a nowhere land of darkness. In such cases, the insomnia is defined as a condition of not being able to get back to sleep. The third type focuses on awakening too early. What to do at 4:00 A.M. or 4:30 A.M. is the major complaint of this type.

Many people have experienced each of these kinds of sleep problems from time to time. However, most people have not had to suffer the ravages of insomnia as a regular diet and so do not really understand the dreadful suffering generated by this problem.

> A 19-year-old male patient who was a college student would have to muffle his screams of rage in his pillow at not being able to get to sleep. He reported that he watched the clock throughout the night—minute by minute and hour after hour. In the morning he would get out of bed exhausted from lack of sleep and frazzled with anxiety, and get ready for his first class beginning at 8:30 A.M. This condition first began when he left home to attend college and it had been occurring intermittently for about two and one-half years.

The separation effect in the onset of this insomnia was relatively easy to trace; work in therapy focused on this person's mixed feelings about leaving home.

> Another patient, a woman in her 50s, awakened after only one or two hours of sleep. She spent the next four or five hours trying to get back to sleep but felt wide awake. Her condition had existed for the past 10 years and may have been triggered

> by her oldest daughter's marriage which occurred sometime before the onset of the insomnia.

The relationship between mother and daughter was especially close; although this woman welcomed her daughter's marriage, it signalled for her a distinct transition, *a leaving* not only of the physical presence of her daughter but also of one stage of her life. She began to feel older and became somewhat depressed.

> Still another patient, a woman in her 30s, developed acute insomnia when she and her husband of one year separated. She was able to fall asleep, but in the wee hours of the morning—about 4:00 A.M.—she would awaken wide-eyed and fully alert. She would obsess about whether her husband would commit suicide over their separation. She would then spend the remainder of the morning until 8:00 A.M. simply obsessing and worrying.

What emerged from this woman's analysis was that she was really quite angry at her husband for making her life so miserable. She blamed him for most of her difficulties and after a while it became clear that her worries with respect to his possible suicide really represented, in a disguised way, an angry wish for his death. When this was clarified and understood in treatment, she began sleeping normally.

Each of these three types of insomnias may be analyzed with respect to several additional factors. For example, it may be necessary to understand the particular factors that constitute pathological or sick insomnia within each of these types. In addition, it may be important to distinguish chronic prolonged insomnia from situational or temporary insomnia (Ware, 1979). Finally, it may become necessary to determine whether a person's report of insomnia is accurate or imagined. In the following section, a review of each of these additional factors will be provided.

THE VALIDITY OF ONE'S INSOMNIA

1. *Insomnia That Is Not Insomnia*—Sometimes individuals claim to

be awake the entire night and swear that they are aware of every minute's passing. However, such claims are only valid in spirit. There is no doubt that many such individuals believe they have been continuously awake. Yet, laboratory studies in sleep research clinics show that they may actually have gotten anywhere from three to five hours of sleep (Hartmann, 1970). Some studies have shown that such persons, when awakened from a dream, will not remember the dream and will deny having slept (Williams and Karacan, 1973). Electroencephalograph (EEG) readings will have indicated that the subject was in fact dreaming and producing REM (rapid eye movement) of dreams. A typical question and answer in a sleep laboratory after the experimenter has just awakened a sleeping subject is:

Q. What has been happening?
A. Nothing. I'm just waiting here.
Q. Have you been to sleep at all?
A. No—not a wink.

Apparently, the patient has complete amnesia for the dream as well as for the amount of time in sleep. The outstanding finding here is the instantaneous amnesiac effect on both the psychological and physiological sense of elapsed time while the patient was actually asleep. This kind of person, though asleep part of the time, usually awakens and feels dreadful. Sleep is not at all remembered and usually such individuals never feel refreshed or rested by whatever actual sleep they did get (Globus, 1970).

Another type of insomniac whose experience of sleeping and wakefulness does not correspond to actual laboratory findings is the one who, surprisingly, reports normal sleep from time to time and actually feels refreshed from this ostensible sleep, even though EEG findings indicate that these persons were actually *not* fully sleeping. This phenomenon is also observed in highly dependent personality types whose dependency needs are being fully gratified but who nevertheless sleep very little; they feel secure, buoyant and rested with whatever minimal sleep they do achieve (Jones and Oswald, 1968; Williams, Karacan and Hirsch, 1974).

2. *Insomnia That Is Temporary*—The kind of insomnia that is likely to be temporary is caused by temporary conditions in a person's life. Acute crises of all kinds may cause this type of insomnia. Frequently, these crises will involve important people in one's life. The emotions generated by such crises include fear of separation, anger over being abandoned, frustration over impeded goals, and feelings of other general loss experiences. What typically occurs as a result of these experiences is that such people sense either a personal depletion of energy or in some instances even an increase in agitation and increased energy. In addition, they may experience a lessening of self-esteem and an overall inability to compensate for whatever insecurities they may feel. When these conditions subside, the insomnia correspondingly dissolves (Williams et al., 1979).

A clear example of the onset and resolution of a case of temporary insomnia is offered by Luce and Segal (1969). A man who had formerly been a good sleeper developed insomnia in response to a temporary situation of separation. The man's wife and oldest daughter were on a trip to France for several weeks.

> "I was taking care of the four children, the dog, the housework—and suddenly I found I was unable to sleep more than an hour and a half at night. Now, I'm a person who likes his eight hours of sleep. Still, I was full of energy. I wasn't tired during the day. I was lonely and maybe I was anxious—I would try to sleep longer but I just had too much energy."

As soon as this man's wife and daughter returned, his insomnia disappeared. It was not the extra work that had caused his insomnia, but rather the *separation* from his wife and daughter. This man's insomnia was not particularly serious because it was temporary and situational. Yet, he did experience it and, even in temporary situations, insomnia, for some, can be terribly anxiety-producing. The question then becomes related not only to insomnia per se, but also to one's significant relationship and its effect on the appearance of insomnia, depression and any other associated symptoms.

3. *Insomnia That Is Dangerous*—The kind of insomnia that is dangerous produces a breakdown of physical and mental processes as a result of actual prolonged lack of sleep (Berger and Oswald, 1962; Kales et al., 1970). Even though certain people may overestimate the amount of time they have not slept, nevertheless many insomniacs do, in fact, become quite ill because of lack of sleep. In certain respects, insomnia is a euphemism for free-floating anxiety—that is, the insomnia is only a symptom of some more serious underlying disorder that can eventually emerge in an unexpected form (Williams et al., 1979). When this more serious problem begins to develop, a person may not even be able to think normally. This kind of thinking problem includes an impairment of concentration and judgment and may develop into a pervasive cognitive impairment. Insomnia begins to signal severe problems whenever such cognitive impairment appears, especially in conjunction with emotional and mental difficulties (Karacan and Williams, 1971).

This severe problem may occur with insomniacs who feel awake throughout the night even though tests show them to be asleep at least some of the time. Yet, those who feel they are awake all of the time can also be accurate with regard to their bodily experiences even though they are inaccurate about their actual sleep experiences. It seems that if a person feels awake all the time, then perhaps even during brief periods of sleep this person's physiology remains heightened. Sleep should be a period of physical, emotional and mental restoration. If someone is in a state of heightened tension *even while asleep,* it is no wonder such persons feel they have not slept. In such cases, breakdowns of all sorts are likely to occur. This is a quite different condition from someone who sleeps approximately the same amount but feels refreshed upon awakening. Feeling refreshed upon awakening even though minimal sleep was achieved means that in certain respects perhaps even minimal sleep can be considered good sleep both emotionally as well as physiologically (Hartmann, 1970). This point shall be fully considered in the following chapter on good and poor sleep.

A STUDY OF SLEEP DEPRIVATION

The untoward psychological effects of sleep deprivation can be vividly seen in an exploration pilot study conducted to measure the effects of sleep deprivation on the performance of various mental and physical tasks. Subjects of the study were a group of firemen who volunteered to participate and to stay awake for various periods of time. Some subjects were deprived of sleep for more than two days.

These subjects were given various motor-performance tasks to complete at various stages of their sleep-deprivation cycle and were also evaluated with psychological tests. The tests that were used to ascertain psychological and emotional changes were designed to measure several functions. First, results on these tests showed the degree of impairment of concentration in these subjects as a function of amount of time they had not slept. As sleep deprivation increased, concentration ability, as would be expected, generally decreased. Second, the tests were able to measure the level or amount of frustration that was experienced as a function of sleep deprivation. Results showed that increased sleep deprivation generated greater and more intense frustration. As a matter of fact, even mild mannered and very proper types became belligerent and, in some cases, even physically threatened those around them. These subjects were exceedingly sensitive to any demands made upon them after they had been sleep-deprived for various periods of time. Third, the sleep-deprived subjects could not easily learn and retain new material. Finally, when asked to solve problems that required use of imagination, a sleep-deprived subject generally relied on magical solutions to problems. For example, when subjects were shown pictures depicting people in conflict, they were unable to provide solutions to these events. Instead, subjects would simply state either that the problem would solve itself or that the story characters "lived happily ever after." Problem-solving ability, the capacity to think about implementing workable solutions to problems, the ability to concentrate, and motivation to work were profoundly impaired in all subjects who were sleep-deprived. Such subjects could only think magically—wishing for something and then expecting it to occur. This kind of thinking reflected immature functioning and dramatically showed the effect of poor sleep on one's mental and emotional capacities.

Of course, the sleep deprivation in this experiment was self-imposed. It must be remembered that these subjects volunteered for the experiment. Nevertheless, the effects of such sleep deprivation on performance of tasks generally and on one's mental health in particular is remarkably similar to the effects produced by actual severe insomnia (Kales et al., 1970). Other studies have shown that sleep deprivation will even produce bizarre psychotic-like behavior. Auditory and visual hallucinations are effects frequently observed in persons who volunteer to participate in sleep-deprivation studies requiring subjects to stay awake for several days (Dement, 1960; Fischgold, Lavernhe and Blanc, 1967).

The associated psychological symptoms of insomnia suggest that it may be connected with other underlying pathological processes that are going on in the person but which are not immediately apparent (Gulevich, Dement and Johnson, 1966; Kales et al., 1969; Kales and Kales, 1973; Sampson, 1966). Sometimes the insomnia is the harbinger of serious mental problems, including suicidal possibilities. In the following chapter, a clinical case illustration will be presented of the appearance of suicidal themes in a woman who had first experienced insomnia six months previously. This is a case of insomnia caused by psychological problems and illustrates Ware's (1979) formulation that a large percent of insomnia is indeed primarily caused specifically by psychological problems and not by interference with sleep mechanisms.

Chapter 10

A Case of Insomnia and the Appearance of Suicidal Thoughts

HOSPITALIZATION

Diane, a 31-year-old woman, was admitted to a state hospital because of emotional and mental problems. Her husband had discovered her lying in the bathtub unconscious. Apparently, she had taken a giant overdose of medication in an attempt to commit suicide. The police were called and she was admitted to the hospital within a few hours. Her stomach was pumped and she was placed on a 90-day observation period.

Diane was somewhat incoherent. She would mumble a few words unintelligibly, was lethargic and unable to concentrate, and cried continuously. Her husband reported that for the past month, and for periods of time before that, she had been frantic, frigid, full of energy, and quite agitated. She would unintentionally shatter glassware and in her frenetic manner would occasionally walk into doors and furniture. In general, she was out of control.

After her suicide attempt she appeared severely depressed and seemed totally demoralized. During the first interview, she could not look directly at the examiner. She was quite tired and could not stop crying. Several events surrounding her suicide attempt required clarification, but she first needed to become less frightened and depressed before she could be fully interviewed.

For the most part, she spent the first few days in the hospital sleeping. She was evidently exhausted because of her ordeal and the new tranquilizing medication she had begun to take. After these first few days, she was scheduled for talks with various hospital personnel and was recommended for psychotherapy as well as for psychological testing and evaluation.

Diane's first week in the hospital, therefore, was one in which she was enabled to regain some semblance of stability. She was seen by several ward personnel who, in an attempt to be supportive, made no demands on her whatsoever. They tried to meet her requests regarding any contacts she may have wanted to have with family and friends. They were also responsive to whatever tensions she had about the hospitalization itself. The first in-depth contact with her occurred during her second week in the hospital.

THE FIRST INTERVIEW

Her mood was gray. She felt hopeless and did not seem to care about anything. Her emotion was flat and she talked in a monotone voice that sounded like a dull hum. She did not want to see her daughters or her husband. Her father who lived in the midwest was not really involved in her life in any substantial way; although he had been notified of her hospitalization, he had not tried to reach her.

She spoke at first in monosyllables, simply answering questions with a defeated "yes" or "no." If asked to elaborate, she seemed able to, but she just could not see the point to it all—as though she felt there was nothing of any value left for her in life. Nevertheless, she gradually began to describe her feelings of despair, her depression, her marriage, and her insomnia. She stuck to the generalities of her life and did not reveal any details of her suicide attempt or of the circumstances leading to her hospitalization.

After some time she admitted that her husband and she were

having marital difficulties. Their sexual relationship had ceased several months earlier because Diane "lost interest." She had been terribly agitated and irritable for several months and was taking large doses of Valium which a friend had given her. During this time she lost all enthusiasm for her job as assistant buyer for a chain discount store and was eventually fired. She simultaneously lost interest in housework and participated only in a perfunctory manner in her children's lives. She attended to only the bare essentials of daily living. She mentioned that she was fond of her husband but could no longer be married to him. She said she never should have gotten married at the age of 19; her choice in a marital partner would be much different at the present time. The interview ended with Diane's deep sigh. She thanked the interviewer for seeing her and asked if he would be by again. Another meeting was then scheduled.

HISTORY

Diane was 31 years old and had recently celebrated her 12th wedding anniversary. Her daughters were 10 and 11 years old. She married her only boyfriend whom she met in high school.

Her mother died of cancer when Diane was 15 and her father could not manage raising his family, which consisted of Diane and an infant son of two. The year Diane married, her father relocated to a small midwestern city. He apparently remarried one year later. She had seen him and her younger brother three times in 12 years. She had never met her stepmother and suspects that this woman would not accompany her father on visits because of some secret issue in their lives. Over the years she has imagined that her father either married a relative or perhaps a woman of another race. Then again, she would dismiss such theories as nonsense and would just wonder about it.

Her mother was an affectionate woman and Diane was devastated by her death. Before she died she told Diane to be happy. Diane's father was unequal to the challenge of supervising a virtually grown daughter and Diane could never count on him for guidance and understanding. She described him as remote and insensitive and said that her mother had often indicated how much in error she was ever to have married him. Her mother had on several occasions warned Diane not to make the same mistake. She told Diane that she was attracted to her father because he was a tall, strong, silent type who, it seemed, would protect her and on whom she felt she could depend. It turned out, however, that this strong silent type was a person whose silence reflected his inability to talk and to relate. He was insensitive and needed continual instruction from Diane's mother about virtually all social expectations. He could not be decisive, was passive and withdrawn, and was generally intimidated by the slightest show of authority. One of the last things Diane's mother told her was to never marry the tall, strong and silent type.

Diane married Peter at the age of 19. He was 26. He was tall, strong and silent. Her sense that she could depend on him was based upon the nature of their social contact in which Peter virtually worshipped her. He would give her anything she wanted and take her anywhere she wanted—mainly because he felt he had to fulfill the needs of others first and because he didn't know where to go or what to do on his own. He never expressed any personal priorities. He could not easily express any personal needs and, according to Diane, never really seemed to have any needs. She said,

> "By the time I was 25 or 26 it was too late. I had two daughters in grade school, a husband who was devoted but who was as immature as a child, and I suddenly realized—oh my God, I've married my father! I did it! All I could do for the next few years, it seemed, was to think about how I'd followed in my mother's path. I did exactly what she told me not to do. I even thought that I, too, would die prematurely."

For the next few years Diane sought help from time to time. She visited several psychotherapists but never returned for a second visit to any of them. She could not improve her marital situation nor could she extricate herself from it. When she was 28, upon the advice of a friend she took a job as a salesperson in a department store. Within one month she was promoted to assistant buyer as an on-the-job trainee. Of course, Peter was agreeable to any plans she had and encouraged her to seek employment. Diane suggested that she knew he really didn't like it because it meant that she would be meeting other men. Peter knew, Diane said, that if she were to leave him, he would have great difficulty keeping any mature woman interested. Diane indicated that because of this fear he really did not want her to work. She said parenthetically that by the time her children were preschoolers she could not bear sexual contact with him.

Indications of insomnia started about the time Diane realized what she considered to be Peter's pathetic, compliant and immature nature. She began to see him as a pudgy overgrown child. Sexual contact became increasingly difficult for her. She became more and more unavailable to him sexually, and at the age of 26 or 27 finally felt sexually frigid whenever they had any contact. She desperately needed to depend on someone who was strong, but felt hopelessly trapped with an ineffectual husband. She masturbated frequently.

SEXUAL PROBLEMS

Diane was a vivacious, attractive and intelligent woman. There was a compelling quality about her and wherever she went, people could depend on her for a stimulating and engaging time. Peter would tag along. Diane was even eloquent at times while Peter spoke mostly in clichés. She was a voracious reader and at about this time, for sexual stimulation, she started reading Victorian sex novels. She had finally found her aphrodisiac. She began to masturbate even more frequently than she previously had. She called this masturbation "compulsive" and said it was reminiscent of her compulsive masturbation during adolescence. Whenever she could, she would turn to her favorite passages in these books and became transformed by their effect on her.

Eventually, she started worrying about her immersion in these fantasies. Whenever she realized her husband wanted sexual contact, she would fantasize some particularly exciting sexual situation as an attempt to become stimulated. These attempts were not entirely successful but they made her contact with Peter more tolerable.

She finally confided her predicament to a friend. In turn, her friend confided a similar predicament and, in addition, confessed that her husband, whom she feared, forced her to act-out fantasies and scenes from pornographic movies and from "dirty books." Her friend described her husband as a strong and generally angry person who needed to act-out very submissive roles in which she would play the role of a dominant slave-mistress. Apparently, this man would need to grovel on the floor and literally needed to be stepped on. This kind of acting-out enabled him to function sexually. Diane was instantly electrified by the entire story and especially by the image of this large man crawling on the floor. She began to think of her own favorite erotically charged stories in which similar themes were portrayed.

From that point on, whenever Diane masturbated she fantasized her friend's husband acting-out his submissive fantasies. Occasionally, she substituted Peter in the fantasy. She could not remember when it happened, but eventually all her masturbatory fantasies were of Peter in a submissive posture while she became his controller. She then would only accede to Peter's sexual advances provided that he did not at first kiss her, did not lie on top of her during sex, and did not embrace her. She would, however, permit him to have oral sex with her. When this occurred, she could then feel sexual and participate more fully. After several months of engaging in this new sexual form, she began telling Peter to perform specific acts and to say certain things to her. It started by her suggesting he say "please." She indicated that usually the thought of sexual contact with Peter would practically anesthetize her. Yet, when she could fantasize acting-out her fantasies, she would become "extremely hot." She reported that at times she even ached to have Peter crawl and grovel at her feet. She eventually confessed her needs to him and he readily entered into her fantasy in a real way.

When Diane began acting-out her fantasies with Peter, she also became depressed. She would agonize over what she considered to be her split-personality. She felt alive during sex and completely alienated from everything at all other times. She detested herself after the sexual contact with Peter, but she could not stop it. Peter felt she finally needed him.

A DEGRADING SEXUAL ACT AND DEPRESSION

Diane finally acted-out her most exciting sexual fantasy. She would expose herself to Peter in seductive ways and at inopportune moments for him. Then she would suggest oral sex in which he would assume a submissive attitude. He would say things to her that indicated just how much he was under her sexual power. This activity continued for some time. It would satisfy her sexual needs but in the aftermath it would depress her badly.

She then suddenly began to want to assume Peter's role of the submissive-slave and for Peter to be the dominant slave-master. They began to act-out this fantasy, after which Diane would become practically disoriented. The thought of acting-out a submissive sexual role with Peter depressed her more severely than ever. At this time she became so despondent that she could not continue to go to work. Once, she even ran out of the house when Peter suggested they "play their game." For the first time, she could not sleep for days on end. She finally consulted a sex therapist and started joint therapy sessions with Peter. The therapist was able to convince them to cease acting-out these fantasies. After one week she was less despondent but still could not sleep. She was given antidepressant medication and diagnosed as having a depressive reaction accompanied by symptoms of insomnia. After only a few meetings, she discontinued all sessions.

Her condition remained at this status for a month or two. She was somewhat depressed but not despondent and she and Peter ceased all sexual activity. She also ceased masturbating. She was able to work consistently but her condition of insomnia was beginning to plague her.

LOVE AFFAIR AND SUICIDE ATTEMPT

Diane became attracted to a salesman who periodically would arrive in town on selling trips. This man lived in another part of the country, was married and was the father of three children. She was a shade over 30 and he was 54. He was sensitive, attractive, considerate and decisive. He wasted no time in approaching her and they began having more contact. They began their affair the day Diane confided her impossible family situation to him.

Diane developed a deep attachment for this man. She said she loved him. He became her magnificent obsession and she desperately wanted to marry him. She felt she had finally found someone who could protect her. During this period, her insomnia was only minimal, her mood shifted, she began to sparkle, and she felt restored. Her misery was becoming a thing of the past.

This hiatus was short-lived. Her friend's phone calls became more limited whereas before they had been frequent. When she called him at his office, she could not always reach him. When she complained to him, he indicated he did not want the kind of pressure she was exerting. He suggested they refrain from any further contact for a while.

Diane was not able to cope with this profound rejection, and became immobilized with anxiety. She began taking large doses of Valium. Within a month her job was terminated, she was in the depths of depression and she was experiencing suicidal thoughts. She could not sleep at all and became frantic. She also could no longer eat to the point of becoming anorectic. In a short time she lost 20 pounds. Her personal health habits also deteriorated. Days and nights seemed to blend and she became extremely agitated.

She remembered wanting to be warm when she died. She filled a tub with hot water, ingested her remaining supply of Valium as well as many aspirin, and got into the bathtub. Her husband found her soon thereafter, asleep but alive. It was at this point that she was hospitalized.

DIAGNOSIS AND PROGNOSIS

In the hospital Diane was diagnosed as a chronic depressive personality with severe insomnia. The extent to which this diagnosis truly reflected her state of mind and her inner conflicts was not clear. What was not questionable was the observation that her particular insomnia was of the dangerous kind that ushers in a pre-psychotic deterioration.

Diane remained in the hospital for almost a year. Unfortunately, her hospitalization was largely a period of convalescence but not therapeutically helpful for correcting her real, underlying psychological problems. She was seen for therapy only irregularly and by a host of temporary hospital staff. When she was released, she was far better than she had been. She was somewhat pessimistic but not apparently depressed. She was taking a regular dosage of antidepressant medication. She made arrangements to live alone and planned to find employment. Then she planned to have her daughters live with her.

Three weeks after being released from the hospital, Diane was dead! A neighbor whom she had apparently befriended indicated that Diane complained of being unable to sleep. She was 32 years old when she was found dead in a tub of cold water. She apparently repeated her original suicide attempt; by the time she was found, the water in the bath was cold. Insomnia was not the cause of her death. Her insomnia was a symptom of a serious mental deterioration which it helped worsen.

This devastating suicide demonstrates how a severe condition of insomnia may transform the complete psychological and emotional structure of a person's life. In this case, the insomnia signalled a pre-psychotic condition and then a profound depressive breakdown. Diane could not reverse this process. Her hospitalization only offered her more time and provided her with a transient sense of security. It temporarily stabilized her, but she could not remain in this sanctuary forever.

Leaving the hospital which had offered her a much needed and satisfactory dependency setting must have represented some sense of significant *separation* to her and it was this separation—reminding her of all previous separations—that triggered a new phase of insomnia, new and flooding feelings of depression, and a commanding sense of doom.

Essentially, her prognosis was bleak from the beginning. She was a severely dependent person with no possibility of obtaining any gratifications. She did not attend therapy sessions regularly—either in or out of the hospital. She changed therapists often and so could not establish a working alliance with any of them. Finally, she developed depression with insomnia—the kind that can kill. Under such unfavorable circumstances it is questionable whether a person like Diane could have been helped, even though her many sterling qualities were evident—they managed to shine through her depressive fog. Her suicide was a tragic end to her life.

Her intense dependency need was painfully exposed when her lover imposed his edict of separation. Her dependency needs and this separation experience—the core ingredients of insomnia—combined to produce the obliteration of sleep because sleep signifies being *with* someone in reality or in fantasy. She was alone in both.

THE ISSUE OF SEPARATION

The true insomniac is in a continual state of dread and guardedness about sleeping. In the vast majority of cases, as illustrated by Diane's experiences, it is highly probable that a person with insomnia is troubled by a breach in an important current relationship, by a difficult past relationship that has been reignited, or by the absence of a relationship. This focus on whole relationships and broken relationships is important because it becomes the central emotional consideration—in the sense of well-being—among people with significant problems in the area of dependency.

The problem with the troubled sleeper is that severe dependency needs require the presence of a significant other person who can satisfy these needs (Bergman, 1971; Bowlby, 1973; Hinton, 1967). Thus, the psychological and symbolic meaning of sleep refers to the existence, either past or present, of a close relationship with a significant person in one's life. Even if a close relationship with another person does not currently exist, the more important issue is whether or not one has ever existed. The more and better the attachments, both past and present, in such persons, the more likely for good sleeping to develop; the fewer and poorer the attachments, both past and present, in such persons, the more likely for poor sleeping to develop. Between these two extreme poles are many significant variations of the nature of attachments.

Separation experiences, therefore, will generally produce sleep problems (Bergman, 1971; Bowlby, 1973; Kupfermann, 1971; Peretz, 1970). As suggested above, these problems are more likely to appear in persons who are inordinately dependent. However, not all people with insomnia are unhappy. If the dependent relationship is generally a well-developed one, so that mutual dependencies exist and each partner is reasonably satisfied, then the one who cannot easily sleep can become occupied during the evening hours with all sorts of activities while the other partner blissfully sleeps away. The mere presence of the sleeping partner in a successful dependent relationship is sometimes enough to permit the poor-sleeping partner an anxiety-free night. This is true even if sleep becomes an on-again, off-again proposition. However, should something unforseen, such as illness or death, occur to the better-sleeping partner, then the one with insomnia may suddenly become tortured for lack of sleep. *The separation effects in people who are inordinately dependent can be severe when their usual support systems are removed.* In a general way, the primary effect of a loss of support may be the appearance of depression. One specific effect of such separation and depression may be the onset of an insomnia condition. This is what occurred in the case of Diane. Good sleep or even poor sleep that is worry-free generally implies the existence, either in the present or in the past, of an intact relationship. This intact relationship may even be neurotic. If it is intact, however, the likelihood of anxious-insomnia developing in one of the partners is small.

Diane's insomnia, of course is not the only kind that exists. It is illustrated here only because it underscores quite clearly the psychological ingredients of a dangerous form of insomnia. Most individuals who experience insomnia can be helped and very often cured. There are other types of insomnias that simply make sleeping more distressing and difficult. Such varieties of insomnia may be better understood through the analysis of those physiological conditions that constitute good sleep and those that generate poor sleep. This issue shall be discussed in the following chapter.

Chapter 11

The Nature of Insomnia: Good Sleep versus Bad Sleep

THERE IS GOOD SLEEP AND BAD SLEEP

Normal sleeping is measured by the appearance of sleep stages in their correct sequence. When people sleep, they quickly enter the first stage. Stage 1 or light sleep is deepened in stage 2 and is followed by stages 3 and 4. The deepest sleep, known as the delta or *D* state, along with REM-dreaming represents one of the most important aspects of normal sleeping. After *D*-sleep in stage 4, one begins to prepare for the dream part of the cycle or the rapid eye movement stage. This cycle of sleep stages and dreaming occurs approximately every 90 minutes (Kleitman, 1970; Hartmann, 1970). Any person who, in a consistent manner, experiences this normal progression of physiological response will not develop insomnia. It is only when some alteration in the sequence of normal stages occurs, or when one of the stages is either over- or underrepresented, that poor sleeping is likely to develop (Agnew, 1964; Hauri and Hawkins, 1973; Monroe, 1967). Under adverse or abnormal sleep cycle conditions, people may begin to experience several different kinds of insomnia.

Studies show that some people who complain about not sleeping at all actually get more sleep than they think. Others, who think they have gotten some sleep, may actually, on the basis of physiological recordings, prove to have gotten less sleep than they think (Williams and Karacan, 1973). Zung (1968) reports that a patient who had a 25-year history of insomnia actually recorded no difficulty in falling asleep and had a normal amount of sleep. Yet this patient kept saying that she "didn't sleep a wink." This phenomenon shall be discussed in the following sections.

Of the average normal sleeper it may be said that 16 percent of sleep is in the *D*-sleep phase while 23 percent of an average normal sleep is in REM or dream-sleep (Hartmann, 1970; Zung, 1970). During each sleep sequence, as long as one fulfills such sleep requirement percentages, sleep disturbance will be at a minimum. It is when these percentages are significantly modified, or when they are not correctly synchronized with the sleep-dream cycle, or when one of of them is absent entirely that sleep problems in the form of insomnia will occur.

BAD SLEEP AND THE SLEEP-DREAM CYCLE

One of the most important discoveries about normal sleeping is that *D*-sleep occurs within the first three hours of the sleep-dream cycle. The point is that difficulty in falling asleep corresponds to a loss of a good portion of *D*-sleep. When loss of *D*-sleep occurs, then people complain of lethargy, a drugged feeling, and generally bad feelings upon awakening (Agnew, Webb and Williams, 1964).

This finding implies that the insomniac who falls asleep relatively easily but awakens several hours later may actually have already experienced the "fruit" of sleep. Such persons may worry about not being able to fall back to sleep and their anxiety can be noxious. Yet, the fact remains that such persons may have gotten enough ***important*** sleep to feel well. In contrast, persons with insomnia who miss *D*-sleep but who will sleep for the remainder of the night can awaken in the morning, and, knowing full well that they slept most of the night, still not be able to explain why they feel exhausted. The answer is that such persons simply may have missed the aspect of the sleep-dream cycle representing the deepest, most restful, and perhaps most restoring part of sleep. It is no wonder that such people feel tired (see Figure 2.1, p. 31).

Those who sleep very little but who believe they have slept more than they actually have are probably getting all of their *D*-sleep and thus may feel refreshed upon awakening. The remainder of sleep beyond *D*-sleep simply does not compare in quality to *D*. In the absence of *D*-sleep and REM sleep, the very serious threat of panic, terror, fury, desperation, and thoughts of suicide will most likely become generated. Most people with insomnia, however, will lose only portions of their *D*-sleep and REM-dream sleep. When monitored in laboratory situations, such subjects are observed to lapse into periods of sleep, but awakening they deny that they were sleeping. When asked to describe the events in the laboratory during the period of time in question, they invariably are at a loss to do so. What this means is that insomniacs generally will underestimate their amount of sleep and correspondingly will overestimate their insomnia. It is the worry and anxiety about loss of sleep, not actual loss of sleep, that usually create in insomniacs feelings of nighttime dread.

Unquestionably, insomniacs use up *D*-sleep quickly and will have poor REM-dream periods. Good sleepers, on the other hand, have good REM and good *D* and have them in the correct sequence.

THE SPECIAL NATURE OF DELTA (D) SLEEP AND REM SLEEP

The *D* state constitutes the single most important sleep state necessary for physiological as well as psychological rejuvenation (Hauri, 1970). If delta time is consistently deprived, one will develop all sorts of physical and bodily symptoms (Agnew, Webb and Williams, 1964; Dement, 1960). In contrast, deprivation of REM-dream activity will generate complaints in subjects of moodiness, depression, lethargy, anxiety and irritability (Dement, 1960; Greenberg, 1967; Hawkins, 1979; Sampson, 1966).

Persons who suffer from the kind of insomnia that is severe usually are the ones who cannot fall asleep easily so that a good deal of early evening delta sleep is interfered with. Furthermore, these persons, upon finally falling asleep, will then experience frequent awakenings. They will sometimes be awakened by the very dreams occurring during REM periods which are necessary to the physical restoration process of the body and to overall emotional well-being. Thus, severe insomniacs are likely to miss some delta sleep and some REM sleep. The extent of this cumulative deprivation can contribute to the nature of potential physical and mental breakdown. REM frequently occurs at the tail end of stage 4 delta sleep or may be considered a separate and distinct period of the sleep cycle (Dement and Mitler, 1973; Hartmann, 1967). The difference between REM and delta sleep as measured by the electroencephalogram (EEG) shows that subjects who are aroused from delta sleep report no dreams while the majority of subjects who are aroused during REM sleep will report dreams.

An interesting finding with respect to delta stage 4 sleep concerns the experience of children who sometimes awaken from this stage sleep with what is called night-terror. When questioned, such children cannot remember dreaming. In contrast, these children, if awakened by a nightmare, will indeed be able to report it. The remembered nightmare, however, was dreamed during REM sleep.

One major difference between each of these stages refers to the state of physiological arousal characterizing them. During deep delta sleep, respiration is slow, heart rate is slow, and most vital signs are in a state of deep relaxation. During REM sleep, respiration, heart rate and other vital physiological processes are heightened.

The pilot study of firemen reported in Chapter 9, who volunteered to stay awake and who showed a whole variety of insomnia associated problems, may be understood as one of primary delta and REM stage deprivation. These subjects were continually complaining of physical disorders—most likely a function of accumulated delta stage 4 sleep deprivation. Furthermore, psychological tests showed a significant decrease in attention span, concentration and overall interest in life among these people. Emotionally, they were irritable and aggressive—symptoms that were caused by the deprivation of REM-dream sleep.

When anti-depressant medication is administered to people who have severe insomnia, they may again begin to dream. Many of these dreams will contain aggressive and hostile themes. Concurrently, aggressive and hostile behavior may then subside even though other stages of sleep may still be deficient. Such persons may then become less irritable. What this means is that when anger is not permitted to emerge in dreams it may be expressed in reality. When it does appear in dreams, then its actual expression is less likely.

The subjective reports of individuals regarding how they feel about their sleep depend to a great extent on whether delta stage 4 sleep as well as REM sleep is disturbed and whether or not such sleep may have been aborted entirely. Good sleep, then, not only consists of a block of uninterrupted sleep but consists primarily of whether sufficient delta and REM sleep were achieved (Hartmann, 1970; Monroe, 1967).

Those people who claim they achieve no sleep are, therefore, simultaneously correct and incorrect. Laboratory studies show that such individuals do from time to time drift off into sleep. An accumulation of such drifting off can equal three or four hours of total intermittent sleep time. Therefore, such persons are incorrect in reporting that they have not slept at all. They are perhaps more significantly correct to say they have not slept at all only if delta and REM sleep was missed. When delta and REM sleep are missed, then even though other sleep was achieved, it is perhaps *in essence* correct to say that one has not slept.

CIRCADIAN RHYTHM AND CHRONOBIOLOGY

People who sleep fewer hours than required for an average night's sleep adjust the portion of time spent in delta stage 4 and in REM sleep. In the first few hours of the night, such persons will increase their total percentages of stage 4 delta sleep and of REM sleep. Globus (1970), in regard to this internal sleep adjustment, believes that sleep is not a series of states but an adaptive homeostatic mechanism of the body. This means that the mechanisms involved in sleep help keep the body healthy. As a mater of fact, laboratory studies as well as subjective experience indicate that too much sleep can be noxious (Baekeland and Hartmann, 1970; Davidson, 1945; Webb, 1970). Sometimes, when people have too much sleep, they feel quite tired and usually regret having slept so long. Some actually find they awaken with runny eyes and nose, headache and depression. The sleep mechanism as a regulatory one may have evolved in order for physical and psychological restoration to occur; this requires a sufficient amount of delta stage 4 sleep and REM-dream sleep (Dement and Mitler, 1973; Kleitman, 1970). In order to normally experience delta stage 4 and REM-dream sleep, one must first traverse stages 1, 2, and 3—a gradual deepening of sleep (Ware, 1979). The normal 90-minute sleep-dream cycle, therefore, will provide time for sleep to deepen until delta stage 4 occurs. This permits the body to experience fullest relaxation. It will also permit enough time for dreams to occur during REM periods so that the necessary physical and mental effects of dreaming may also have time to develop. The normal sequence of sleep stages reflects an aspect of the body's circadian rhythm. It is an aspect of the temporal nature of biological activity and is part of the study of chronobiology.

Figure 11.1 presents a sample EEG tracing of the state of wakefulness, REM sleep, and the 4 stages of non-REM sleep. These stages are regular rhythmic occurrences of the body and are similar to other chronobiological phenomena.

Dement (1972) describes this figure as follows:

"This figure shows sample EEG tracings which illustrate the typical patterns seen in wakefulness, the four NREM EEG stages, and REM sleep. The top five lines represent thirty seconds of brain wave recording while the bottom line is eight seconds. All were recorded at the standard chart speed of 10 millimeters per second. A 10-millimeter deflection of the recording pen up or down represents a potential change in the brain of about 50 millionths of a volt (microvolts). The first line shows the normal brain wave pattern of relaxed wakefulness. Note the presence of an almost continuous, relatively fast sinusoidal rhythm. This is the well-known alpha rhythm whose fluctuations are characteristically close to 10 cycles

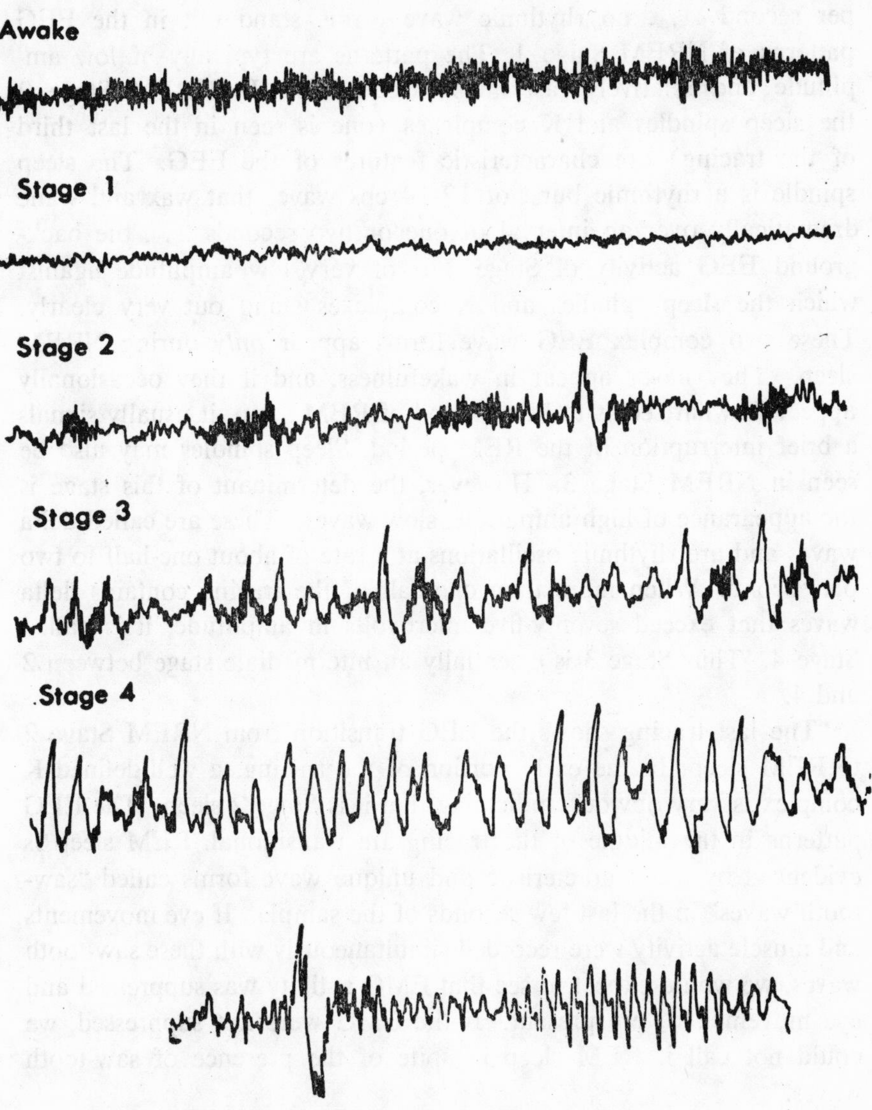

FIGURE 11.1: EEG tracings of the state of wakefulness, REM sleep, and the 4 stages of non-REM sleep. (From: Dement, W. C. *Some must watch while some must sleep*, with the permission of W. W. Norton & Company, Inc. Copyright © 1972, 1974, 1976 by William C. Dement. Originally published as part of the Portable Stanford series by the Stanford Alumni Association, Stanford, Ca.)

per second . . . no rhythmic wave forms stand out in the EEG patterns of NREM Stage 1. The patterns are typically of low amplitude and relatively fast mixed frequencies. In NREM Stage 2 the sleep spindles and K complexes (one is seen in the last third of the tracing) are characteristic features of the EEG. The sleep spindle is a rhythmic burst of 12-14 cps waves that wax and wane dramatically over an interval of one or two seconds . . . the background EEG activity of Stage 2 is of very low amplitude against which the sleep spindles and K complexes stand out very clearly. These two complex EEG wave forms appear *only* during NREM sleep. They never appear in wakefulness, and if they occasionally appear in what seems to be a period of REM sleep, it usually signals a brief interruption of the REM period. Sleep spindles may also be seen in NREM Stage 3. However, the determinant of this stage is the appearance of high amplitude, slow waves. These are called delta waves and are rhythmic oscillations at a rate of about one-half to two per second. When more than one-half of the tracing contains delta waves that exceed seventy-five microvolts in amplitude, it is called Stage 4. Thus Stage 3 is essentially an intermediate stage between 2 and 4.

"The last tracing shows the EEG transition from NREM Stage 2 to REM sleep. In the early portion of the tracing, a well-defined K complex is very obvious, indicating that it is Stage 2 sleep. The EEG patterns in the middle of the tracing are transitional. REM sleep is evidenced by the characteristic and unique wave forms called "saw-tooth waves" in the last few seconds of the sample. If eye movements and muscle activity were recorded simultaneously with these saw-tooth waves, we would expect to see that EMG activity was suppressed and eye movements were present. If the EMG were not suppressed, we could not call it REM sleep in spite of the presence of saw-tooth waves."

Zung (1970) has proposed that the 90-minute sleep-dream cycle, characterized by these sleep stages, is part of a primitive defense against hostile environments, a point also discussed in Part 1 of this book. The sleep mechanism, therefore, may have developed in evolution as an adaptive device to enable a person to quickly gather deep restorative sleep as well as to drift from light to deep sleep and back again. Such a cycle implies a residual evolutionary mechanism of survival expressed in the biological organization of sleep; that is, the sleep cycle contains a process of rising and falling depths of sleep that may have been necessary in development to ensure self-protective and survival needs. This point also underlies the issue of circadian body rhythm referred to in Chapter 6. The regular rhythm of rest and activity known as the Basic Rest-Activity Cycle (BRAC) (Thayer, 1967) is one aspect of the body's rhythm. Similar rhythms of hormonal activity are reported by Halberg (1972), and a whole host of chemical and physiological activities based upon chronobiological function are reported by Mills (1966). Even tumor growth and treatment contain chronobiological properties (Gupta and Deka, 1975).

There is also a growing body of literature that shows the relation between circadian clock impairment (such as a breakdown in stage 4 sleep or in REM dreaming) and the appearance of many bodily disturbances. For example, Stroebel (1968) showed that when rhesus monkeys could not establish regular circadian controls, disturbances such as high blood pressure, reduction in grooming, and asthmatic attacks occurred. The 24-hour wake-sleep rhythm has also been elaborated by Weitzman (1976) and Weitzman, Boyar, Kapen and Hellman (1975) with respect to neuroendocrine function, and by Baldy-Moulinier, Arguner and Besset (1976).

The various forms of insomnia now may be better understood. They are all caused by an irregularity of the process of sleep stages. Thus it is possible to understand the varieties of disordered sleep by knowing the physiological sleep processes that constitute normal sleeping. In order for sleep to be normal, it must go through a normal sequence of stages and should comprise a normal sleep-dream cycle. Disordered sleep refers to interferences of sequence of sleep stages and of dream cycles. Such disorders eventually crystallize as variations of insomnia. In terms of usual insomnia variations, disordered sleep is characterized in three basic ways, as presented in the following section. This division of insomnia-related disordered sleep is also provided by Luce and Segal (1969).

VARIATIONS OF INSOMNIA

Falling asleep itself is the first major problem of insomnia. This is the kind of insomnia that is experienced as torturous: "I just lie there and lie there wide awake," is the frequent description of this type of insomnia. This problem is likely to be serious because delta sleep, as well as REM sleep, may become quite abbreviated. Persons of this type are the ones who complain of never getting any sleep.

The second type of insomnia is one in which multiple awakenings occur. People who experience this problem are likely to have disordered delta and REM sleep, or may not have normal sequential experiences of sleep stages. Stages of sleep in this kind of insomnia may develop in ways that are too long or too short. Furthermore, cycles may be abnormal and REM sleep can also be either too short or abnormally long. Delta sleep is similarly likely to be disturbed.

The third type of sleep—early morning awakenings—may reflect poor sleep, but this kind of insomnia is surely not as problematic as the first two. It is likely that delta and REM sleep are largely achieved in this kind of insomnia. Such insomnia, however, also interferes with the sleep-dream cycle and people who typically experience early morning awakenings report that they are fatigued by mid-afternoon.

The different problems of insomnia are summarized by their relation to delta and REM sleep and to the sequence of sleep-dream cycles. Delta sleep may be too long or abbreviated. The same is true for REM sleep. Cycles may be disordered, and any one of the four sleep stages may be similarly too long or abbreviated. Furthermore, nightmares or even the night-terrors of stage 4 sleep can cause insomnia. In the ordering of these sleep mechanisms it is now possible to understand why people who sleep a lot may not feel rested or why someone may experience a chronic inability to sleep and yet not break down mentally or physically. It is now also possible to understand that people may feel good about their sleep even though they actually sleep only three or four hours each night (Jones and Oswald, 1968). Again, the solution to the puzzle of disordered sleep lies in how much delta and REM sleep was achieved and in how the sequence of sleep stages was experienced. The question of whether the amount of delta and REM sleep as a basic physiological requirement remains constant with advancing age will be examined in the following section with respect to the experience of insomnia throughout life.

DELTA SLEEP AND AGING

Kahn (1970) reports on a number of investigations in which the nature of delta sleep has consistently changed as a function of the aging process. The delta sleep of children is protracted and its duration as part of the sleep cycle decreases as one gets older. Delta sleep continues to decrease in later life. In the very elderly, delta sleep may be quite low. Furthermore, the duration of each stage of sleep has been found also to be decreased so that the onset of REM occurs much sooner as measured from the moment one begins to enter stage 1 sleep.

Kahn proposes that REM will appear sooner than usual in the elderly, primarily because of the abbreviated form of delta sleep in the entire sleep cycle.

One implication of this change in delta sleep in the aged is the prediction that insomnia-like conditions may become a typical experience of elderly people. Elderly people may find it difficult to want to go to sleep early in the evening because of more than one or two naps that they have had during the day. This late getting to sleep, however, predisposes one to a reduction of delta sleep.

Table 11.1 presents sleep stage percentages for age groups showing the reduction in stage 4 sleep as a function of age.

The aging process thus produces insomnia-like wakefulness experiences; from adulthood onward, wakefulness, or a tendency towards wakefulness, becomes a more typical aspect of sleep. It is generally known, that during childhood it is far more difficult to get up during the night even when awakened. All individuals obviously experi-

TABLE 11.1

Sleep Stage Percentages for Age Groupings
(showing the reduction in stage 4 sleep with age)

Age of Group (Years)	Stages of Sleep 1	2	3	4	REM	Mean Sleep Length (Minutes)
21-31 months	8	43	–	18	29	596
8-11	6	44	6	18	24	565
16-19	5	47	6	18	23	454
20-29 (m)	5	50	7	13	24	418
20-29 (f)	6	48	7	16	22	451
30-39	8	53	5	10	22	443
50-59	11	51	8	3	23	436
60-69	12	51	5	3	20	440

(Adapted from: Webb, W. B., and Agnew, H. W., Jr., Measurement and characteristics of nocturnal sleep. In: Abt, L. A., and Riess, B. F. (Eds.), *Progress in clinical psychology,* Vol. 8, New York: Grune & Stratton, 1969.)

ence the powerful effect of delta sleep during childhood even though no one actually knew what it was that caused such a sleep-drugged condition. By contrast, getting out of bed at any time during the night is far easier for adults. In fact, some people prefer to rise once or twice during the night.

> A patient once reported that rising in the middle of the night, when it was peaceful and quiet, gave him a very tranquil feeling, and, further, made him feel that he was, without a doubt, in full control of his life. This man grew up feeling compelled to follow convention and custom in every detail. Sleeping in an obedient fashion—which meant sleeping through the night—was an example of following customs and expectations required of him as a child. When, because of his age, his sleep was no longer a full night of unconscious slumber, he would rise in the middle of the night and begin to feel quite liberated. He would look forward to such awakenings. They would allow him to saunter through the house, just casually looking around. He would sit in a chair in the dark and think to himself, "Ha, this is great." He would then fall off to sleep again.

Of course, this man's wakefulness was not in any way a variation of insomnia. Wakefulness does not only mean insomnia. Insomnia is a clinical condition. It is problematic because it causes anxiety, irritability, or other more serious clinical physical symptoms. Increased age simply has an effect on the sleep cycle (Mendels and Hawkins, 1967; Webb, 1970). Wakefulness becomes a typical aspect and effect of the normal changes in sleep cycles and sleep stages as one ages. Yet, total sleep time may not at all be decreased as age increases. What this means is that people who are older spend more time trying to produce the same amount of sleep than younger people achieve in less time.

As a matter of interest, those who suffer from deprivation of sufficient delta stage 4 sleep have complaints about sleeping similar to those made by the elderly. These complaints concern not being able to sleep and experiencing bodily discomforts, aches and pains, and an overall malaise. It is possible that in the very old delta sleep may be entirely eliminated. There are many implications of this finding, not the least of which is the possibility that an end to delta stage 4 sleep is a harbinger of the end to life itself.

The effect of decreased delta sleep in the elderly is remembered fondly, time and again, by persons who were raised in a household with a grandparent. People who have had this experience will most likely remember the midnight and even night-long persistent prowl, that went from the grandparent's room to the kitchen and back; then to the bathroom and back—ever shuffling through the house and lending to the family, and especially to the children, a 24-hour simultaneously disquieting and comforting presence.

In the following section, a discussion of *sleep apnea,* an axiomatic insomnia condition, and a frightening irregularity of sleep, will be presented.

SLEEP APNEA

Sleep apnea is essentially a sleep respiratory problem (Guilleminault and Dement, 1978). Persons actually stop breathing while asleep and suddenly awaken in order to continue breathing. It is a snoring symptom characterized by gasping-type snoring that can continue all through the night. It can completely disrupt the entire sleep-dream cycle, including the all-important stage 4 delta sleep as well as REM-dream sleep (Gulleminault, Eldridge and Dement, 1973).

Apneas were first reported in 1965. They are frequently reported in persons who smoke heavily and are obese. They are caused by a brain dysfunction related to respiratory regulation. During the sleep apnea, oxygen falls and carbon dioxide rises in the blood. This condition can cause serious cardiovascular problems such as strokes, heart attacks, or high blood pressure. Because of such problems, sleep apnea can also cause death.

Derman and Karacan (1979) define the apnea as a cessation of breathing and present three variations of this problem.

(1) *Central Sleep Apnea*—This type of apnea is characterized by a cessation of breathing for more than 10 seconds. All respiratory activity seems to be suspended during this period of time.

(2) *Obstructive Sleep Apnea*—In this type of apnea, breathing through the mouth and/or nose is suspended but muscle activity in the respiratory service is not; the muscle effort finally undermines the breathing obstruction and breathing will begin. An interesting paradox here concerns the diagnosis of obstructive apnea as both a disorder of initiating and maintaining sleep (DIMS) as well as a disorder of excessive somnolence (DOES). Thus, this disorder is an insomnia condition, but because the subject is always sleepy it can also be considered as a disorder of excessive sleepiness.

(3) *Mixed Sleep Apnea*—This kind of apnea starts as a central sleep apnea and evolves into an obstructive episode. The apnea is overcome by increased muscle effort.

It is conservatively estimated that there are about 50,000 sleep apnea victims in the United States. The disorder can be easily diagnosed if 30 or more episodes occur within a seven-hour period in which each episode lasts more than 10 seconds (Derman and Karacan, 1979).

The sleep apnea is a special disorder of sleeping and its insomnia effect is a virtual equivalent of its actual behavioral effect—that is, breaking through the apneic episode frequently means becoming momentarily awakened. Lugaresi et al. (1976) also discuss the issue of hypersomnia with periodic apnea. The gasp for air is jarring and can keep a person in a continual state of awakening throughout the night.

In the following chapter, the question of the relationship between one's diagnosis and the extent to which such a diagnosis implies an increase in the likelihood of insomnia symptoms appearing will be considered.

Chapter 12

Diagnostic Implications of Insomnia

DO INSOMNIACS SHARE A COMMON PERSONALITY STRUCTURE?

In Part II of this book, depressive and paranoid character traits were attributed to the personality structure of narcoleptics who were chiefly characterized as dependent. The paranoid part of their diagnosis was theorized to be composed of stubborn attitudes, an oppositional tendency, an underlying store of anger, and a severely sarcastic and critical stance towards the world. Yet, it was also proposed that beneath this seemingly impenetrable wall of depression and sarcasm was a nature quite vulnerable and susceptible to all sorts of authority influences. The personality structure of the hysterical person, who may so easily be hypnotized, was identified as the basis for this underlying structure of the narcoleptic. In other words, it was suggested that the narcoleptic who is dependent is a person who needs to appear unreachable because intense feelings of vulnerability prevail beneath the surface.

The opposite formulation is here proposed to reveal the personality of the chiefly dependent person with insomnia. Of course, persons with insomnia can be quite different from one another. Yet common personality ingredients are shared by most sufferers of insomnia who are dependent types whether the insomnia consists of the inability to fall asleep or of awakening several times after sleeping

(Beulter, Thornby and Karacan, 1978). The connective underpinning that can trigger insomnia in such persons is the excessive effect of separation experiences.

People with insomnia are described in the literature on sleep as frantic types—those who worry about phantom problems. Insomnia sufferers insist that they do not sleep, while others tell them that they do and not to worry about it. Insomniacs are described as manic—high energy types—even though the insomnia symptom itself is frequently expressed as a feature of depression (Hinton, 1963). The observation that insomniacs generally are in a higher state of arousal—accompanied by higher temperature and faster respiration and heartbeat—than normal sleepers contributes to the image of the insomniac as a person with an hysterical and frantic personality.

> Helen, a woman in her 30s, finally sought psychotherapy treatment because she claimed that she had not been able to sleep for years. She had recently met a man whom she admired and who she knew was also interested in her. Yet she was terribly frightened by the prospect of marriage and this situation precipitated her current anxiety. Despite her fear of remaining single, she was unable to deepen any relationship of which she was part; because of this inability, she was not free to marry.
>
> Helen was exceedingly concerned with her appearance and would spend inordinate amounts of time gazing into mirrors. Each detail of her dress and facial make-up was perfectly completed; she could not allow herself any measure of imperfection. In addition, she was tense with respect to all sorts of bodily functions. She experienced such a wide array of anxieties that she even laughed at what she said was the absurdity of it all.

This woman's personality structure reflected hysterical as well as anxiety features. Yet, her particular style of coping and her history suggested that beneath her anxiety and hysteria existed an impervious obsessive and paranoid-like streak. She only *appeared* to be influenced by everything and everyone around her, but her history showed that she behaved fundamentally with her own rigid and hidden agenda. This private agenda kept her isolated and separate and contained a highly critical attitude toward the world. She would not allow herself any imperfections and yet she considered the rest of the world as quite imperfect.

> After several sessions, Helen revealed her main obsessive fear. This fear consisted of anticipating the feeling of terror at the prospect of her mother's death. Several years before, her mother became ill and almost died. This event was the pivotal situation from which her symptom of insomnia developed.
>
> The symptom of insomnia reflected the fear of impending separation in this highly dependent woman. She developed hysterical anxiety, and phobic symptoms in response to this potential separation; however, beneath the surface it seemed more as if she felt paranoid, and stubbornly rigid. There were times when she would not leave her house for days.

The personality structure of this woman with insomnia, therefore, seemed to be composed of hysterical anxiety features above and paranoid withdrawal features underneath—diagnostically quite the opposite picture to that proposed for the narcoleptic.

Both the dependent person with narcolepsy as well as the one with insomnia are likely to have developed their respective sleep disorders during some event that was characterized by separation; they are both also presumed to harbor strong depressive feelings. It is further proposed that the key feature of the personality structure of this sort of insomniac is an underlying paranoid-rigid personality. The dependent person with insomnia may be a compulsive type or an energetic manic one, or for that matter may show a multitude of personality features. Yet, it is proposed that the basic underlying personality structure will be unyielding and rigid.

THE MAIN EMOTION OF INSOMNIA

It has been indicated that the main emotion of narcolepsy is the narcoleptic's underlying *fear* of being overcontrolled or influenced by external authority pressure. It is now proposed that the main emotion of insomnia is the insomniac's underlying *anger* at the imperfections in the world, at not being attended to, and at any impending separation from the person on whom they are dependent. As narcolepsy is behaviorally opposite to insomnia, so too is the underlying emotion of fear that is characteristic of the dependent narcoleptic's personality opposite to the emotion of anger that is characteristic of the dependent insomniac's personality. The emotions of fear and anger can produce feelings of alienation and both such feelings can keep one awake or put one to sleep.

The anger inherent in insomnia-related dependent personalities becomes expressed in many ways; for example, insomniacs will frequently undermine their medication regimens by manipulating their drug dosages. They do this contrary to the physician's persistent recommendations to refrain from changing these medication dosages. Such an act reveals the rigidly controlled aim of this kind of person, which is to resist feeling compliant. Parenthetically, this sort of angry resistance against giving in may be seen during arguments between husbands and wives. One or both partners may just lie in bed fuming, not sleeping but also not talking. The way in which such anger and depression become characteristic of insomnia will be considered in the following section.

INSOMNIA AND DEPRESSION: SIX TYPES

Insomnia as a symptom of psychological conflict (Kales et al., 1972; Karacan and Williams, 1971) and change in mood (Kales, Caldwell, Preston et al., 1976) emerges most clearly as an expression of depression (Hinton, 1963; Kales and Kales, 1973). Depressions may occur from a variety of causes—yet virtually all such causes may be classified roughly into six categories. Along with insomnia, sexual dysfunction is also a frequent symptom of all forms of depression.

(1) *Chronic Depression with Insomnia*: This kind of depression is more or less lifelong and is termed *endogenous depression* (Pflug and Tolle, 1971a, b). Persons who suffer this kind of depression are usually fatalistic. They find it difficult to be jubilant or optimistic, even when they are actively engaged in useful projects or activities that they do indeed seem to enjoy. Sometimes such individuals appear to have made a vow never to reveal any shred of optimism—as though to

be happy is to unwillingly offer others the satisfaction of witnessing such moments of enjoyment. With furrowed brow and sobering look, such people evoke a sense of discomfort in those around them. In chronic depression, insomnia is sometimes a serious problem because it may reflect deep underlying suicidal feelings. Kellerman (1976) describes one such case, in which insomnia preceded a suicidal act.

> A 55-year-old man who had been depressed since his teenage years would periodically exhibit a sudden intensification of his depression. During such depressive episodes, his insomnia would keep him awake for days at a time. His family would be alert to any suicidal gestures at times like these. After a while he would just as suddenly seem to feel better; when his depression lifted, family members tended to breathe a sigh of relief and reduce their collective guard.
>
> Unfortunately, the greatest suicidal danger exists when depressive persons with insomnia suddenly, and with no drug intervention, declare that their depression is cured, insomnia has disappeared, and they feel generally wonderful. Instead of reducing their collective vigilance, the family should be even more guarded during these seemingly miraculous and sudden recoveries. In the case described the family believed that this man was improved and they reduced the amount of supervision they had been giving him. At the first chance, he shut all the windows in the house, turned on the gas jets, and committed suicide.

Thus, a person with a chronic depression will probably develop periods of insomnia. These episodes of insomnia—if prolonged—can be a sign of serious suicidal ruminations and fantasies. In this sort of endogenous chronic state, the onset of insomnia, as well as more serious depressive moods, is a common occurrence from time to time. There will always be some pivotal event that triggers any immediate intensified depression and it is frequently useful to try to understand what it was that stimulated this new, and more intense, mood.

> In the case of this man who was a lifelong depressive type, any plans for vacation could upset him. He felt more or less stable when at home and would dread abrupt changes in his

daily routine. He actually liked vacations, but the plans and arrangements necessary to organize any trip positively depressed him. He just could not tolerate attention to the mountain of detail that was necessary at such times.

He had been hospitalized several times over the years, always with the complaint of insomnia, severe depression, and suicidal thoughts. His last case of insomnia and depression was, it seems, caused by the plans his family had to move to a new home 1500 miles away. The family decided that a warm climate, among other reasons, would be more pleasant for him and for them. Unfortunately, this plan started an emotional chain reaction ultimately leading to his death. The planned move represented a deep *separation* to this man—one that he could not emotionally and psychologically manage. Actually such persons are terribly afraid of separations but tend to deny their separation anxieties and substitute sudden flight into health expressions for them. This man did just that; his anxiety was transformed into feelings of well being that ultimately led to his suicide when the family controls were reduced.

(2) *Acute Depression with Insomnia*: Acute depression differs from the chronic kind in that it develops out of some recent traumatic event, such as the death of a loved one. During such experiences, the depression that emerges reflects whatever loss or traumatic experience exists. In addition, acute depressions serve to allay any intense anxiety generated from such traumatic events. In this respect, acute depression is called *reactive depression* to reflect the fact that it is a reaction to a current experience. Its appearance always implies that there is an existing, but hidden, reservoir of intense anxiety.

Insomnia also frequently accompanies this kind of depression but is inhibited by the high doses of sleep medication usually prescribed for people who are so depressed (Kales et al., 1977; Oswald, 1968; Oswald and Priest, 1965). If the depression does not improve, insomnia becomes the chief complaint of people who suffer with this problem.

An 85-year-old man was referred for consultation because of excruciating feelings of depression and a sudden inability to sleep. This sturdy senior citizen reported that he had always been a good sleeper but for the past two months had been both unable to sleep and unable to work. Despite his age, he was employed as a full-time shoemaker in a small shop. He was a vigorous person who appeared to be 10 or 15 years younger than he actually was. He was a widower for the past 25 years, although some time after his wife's death he met a woman with whom he had lived ever since. He reported that his sexual activity had only recently become problematic.

Apparently this gentleman enjoyed a relatively active sex life—one of the best aspects of his relationship with his common-law wife. His insomnia, his impotence, and his depression all occurred at about the same time—two months earlier.

The most immediate therapeutic task with this man was to help him eliminate these severe symptoms and thus give him at least some temporary relief. To do this, it became imperative for him to see that his symptoms were most likely caused by a single specific event involving another person. The point to make was that this kind of depression and its associated symptoms did not occur randomly—that they were connected to events and to people. This elderly patient then confided that just before his symptoms appeared he had visited his eldest son and requested a small loan. He was summarily turned down and instantly felt humiliated—an emotion that can be one of the most powerful in the experience of psychological pain, in the onset of depression, in the suppression of sexual feelings, and in the development of angry feelings. It was difficult for this man even to recount the painful event. He looked away when describing his humiliation, and, in order to soften the experience, excused his son's response by stating how he realized his son had "lots of expenses."

He was asked whether he would consent to a joint session—meeting together with his son. He immediately rejected the idea. The matter was pursued and he eventually agreed to the meeting.

His son, a cardiologist, was quite willing to discuss his father's condition. He was actually very concerned about his father and volunteered the information that he thought his father's depression was caused by their difficult talk regarding the loan. His son felt terribly regretful and wanted to know how to go about repairing the situation. He would gladly offer his father whatever monies his father needed, but he knew that it would now not be accepted. He wanted to tell his father that he looked forward to a joint meeting, that he would do anything to help, and that his angry and impulsive response to the loan request was based upon his preoccupation with other difficulties in his life.

When the message of reconciliation was reported to him, this elderly gentleman became visibly moved. He said that the joint session was not really necessary because his son was a very busy person. Father and son were reconciled soon thereafter. Within several days the symptoms of insomnia and impotence had disappeared and this man returned to work. His therapy visits ended. They had lasted a total of three weeks in which he attended exactly six sessions.

The main issue in this short-term treatment was to locate the pivotal traumatic event from which depression, insomnia, and impotence had arisen. Once identified, the powerful emotion of humiliation could be ventilated and discussed, and a plan could be designed to nullify the noxious event. Of course there were other psychological features of this man's personality that could have been analyzed further. Humiliation is not a pleasant experience. Yet, some will be more sensitive to it than are others. There are those who even can be humiliated at the slightest hint of rejection and then develop depressive symptoms along with insomnia.

This kind of personality feature was not analyzed within the short-term contact. Considering the presenting problem, as well as his age, it was a courageous step in the first place for this man to seek psychotherapy consultation and he did quite well indeed.

(3) *Depression Connected with Hormonal Changes*: There are insomnias that occur because of hormonal problems. The most typical of these occurs in women who, several days before menstruation, may begin to feel tense and experience intermittent bouts of insomnia. Statistics also indicate that poor sleeping is far more prevalent in women than in men. The reason for this difference may, at least in part, be due to monthy hormonal changes based upon menstruation. Such hormonal changes frequently cause increased tension, which in

turn may create an uncomfortable feeling of something impending, depressive feelings, and symptoms of insomnia.

> A young woman of 30 had a history of intense depressive feelings starting several days before the onset of her period. She needed to be on a mild tranquilizer because of it and she hated and dreaded the few days preceding her period.
>
> This woman was also usually quite tense, defensive and guarded. She was inordinately concerned about anyone besting her. She was highly competitive, yet she could not assert herself in a mature way. Her relationships with other women were always competitive and generally unsuccessful. These competitive and immature concerns were readily transparent and most people could not easily tolerate her tensions and her immaturity. She was a person who needed a great deal of reassurance from those around her. Any display of friendship from others would arouse an overburst of enthusiasm in her and an expression of deep appreciation with respect to such approval. This kind of behavior made it difficult for anyone to be close to her. Either she would be devastated by some mild criticism or she would be effusive at some innocuous positive expression of support.

This woman's anxiety and tension-filled expectations centering around her impending period each month were not just a function of physical and emotional effects of hormonal changes. Her reaction to her period was partly psychological. She was the kind of person who, because of deeply-etched inferiority feelings, as well as strong competitive urges, could not permit anyone or anything to control her. The arrival of her monthly period was obviously something she did not design and had no control over. It was going to occur whether she liked it or not.

It was this inexorable quality to her period that made it such a difficult event for her to accept. Several days before it appeared each month, her feelings of anger would soar. She was usually an irritable person to start off with. The arrival of her period would dramatically increase her overall level of anger and would significantly decrease her ability to tolerate any frustrations. The increased level of anger and her sense of personal fragility seemed to generate despairing feelings. Whenever this occurred, she would experience several days of insomnia in which she would have difficulty falling asleep. She described it as a feeling of lying in bed with her fists clenched, in a state of high anxiety.

> In the therapy sessions, she devoted many hours to expressing age-old feelings about her dependence during childhood, her sense of being different from other children her own age, her parents' inordinate and competitively-based expectations of her, and her inability to establish an open, direct and honest relationship with a man. She desperately needed to have an intimate and trusting relationship but seemed unable to find one. Gradually, as she began to analyze her difficulties, she became less fearful. For the first time in her life she became more conscious of her problems and their causes and began to utilize these insights in everyday interactions. Her depressive and angry mood began to lift. In addition, as her inferiority feelings became expressed through the therapy, changes in her behavior ensued. She started feeling more mature. After some months, her insomnia finally disappeared. Even though her periods were still difficult, they became significantly less problematic. She was able to tolerate them without feeling she was being forced to have them against her will.

(4) *Drug Withdrawal Depressions with Insomnia*: A special kind of depression is caused by the abrupt cessation of using drugs (Cooper, 1977; Kales, Bixler, Tan et al., 1974; Kales and Kales, 1970). Insomniacs, narcoleptics, phobic people, and generally depressed people have a tendency to begin to rely on drugs in order to sleep normally and to alleviate the symptoms of depression.

> James, a man in his 40s, was on a regular regimen of antidepressant medication as well as sleep medication. He had been taking this medication continuously for about 10 years. When asked what it was that started him on this regimen of medication, he hesitated for a few moments and said that it had started so long ago that he couldn't quite remember. He vaguely thought the medication was recommended by a physician because of pains in his stomach. He remembered that "the doctor" pre-

scribed the medication as a preventative measure against possible ulcers. In any event, he never returned to this physician and quite on his own had been continuing to take this medication for the past decade.

He was referred for therapy by a former patient—a friend of his—who casually observed him popping pills and smoking marijuana. This friend was astounded at this inordinate need for medication. He suggested to him that the marijuana should have been enough to relax him, and actually convinced him to give up taking the medication.

James did just that; he simply stopped taking his medication. He soon became irritable and moody, had spells of sweating, could not sleep and became depressed. It took him several more days to realize what had happened and he quickly resumed his regimen of medication.

This man developed insomnia and depression as withdrawal symptoms. This is similar to withdrawal states observed with alcoholics and drug addicts. As a matter of fact, this patient had unknowingly become an addict on small doses of anti-depressant and sleep medication. He eventually was able to discard his drugs, but this occurred gradually over several months. His withdrawal symptoms became terrifying when he began having nightmares in which he felt he was choking and drowning. He felt as though he were going to die.

These withdrawal symptoms reflected the fact that his use of drugs and the euphoric feeling of well-being they generated had begun to assume a *compensatory* role in his life, becoming a substitute for a naturally experienced healthy self-image. When he stopped taking his medication, he began to feel weak, depressed, inferior, and without any *compensations* of strength or high self-esteem. Thus, he actually felt he was dying. The gradual withdrawal from medication was the only way he could manage to minimize the potentially crushing symptoms of withdrawing "cold turkey."

(5) *Depressions with Insomnia Caused by Organic Brain Changes*: It is not uncommon to hear stories of elderly people disappearing for days at a time, only to return home and claim not to know where they had been. This kind of event is called *night wandering*. It most

often occurs when some organic damage affects the brain or when, because of arteriosclerotic changes, people begin to behave strangely. Such damage generally indicates that a deterioration of functioning is to be expected in many areas.

> A woman in her 70s, who all of her life had been a dedicated family person, suddenly disappeared from home. She reappeared the following day, embarrassed about not remembering her whereabouts. She was a Chinese woman who had never before been away from home. She was a devoted mother of three and grandmother of six; her sudden disappearance caused panic throughout her immediate and extended family. A neurological examination revealed distinct organic brain changes. Her family reported that for several weeks before her disappearance she had become forgetful, felt depressed and could not sleep at all.

This woman was placed on medication but her prognosis was poor and the family was warned that her condition would deteriorate to the point where she would have to be permanently hospitalized. It is apparent from this case that even in people with organic brain changes, depression and insomnia may appear simultaneously.

Persons with *sleep apnea*—awakenings throughout the night due to malfunction of the brain's respiration regulatory signal—can also experience depression along with this organic insomnia.

(6) *Manic-Depression with Insomnia*: A severe kind of depression, in which intense insomnia appears as a major symptom is that seen in the disorder of manic-depression. This disorder occurs in a phasic manner. A person may be highly energized first, involved in a spate of projects, sleep only about three or four hours per night and become impossibly talkative. This phase may last for several months and then be suddenly transformed into severe depression. The depressive phase will then also last for several months. One of the early signs of the transformation of mania into depression is the complaint of feeling tired because of lack of sleep. Insomnia, therefore, is one of the first signals of an impending depression in this manic-depressive syndrome. A person in the manic phase will frequently be afflicted with sleep onset insomnia and short sleep, while in the depressive phase, although

there is a reasonably good ability to fall asleep, difficulties arise in maintaining sleep and in early morning awakenings.

> An intensely manic woman of 40 was admitted to a state hospital because her inappropriate behavior made her potentially dangerous to herself and to those around her.
>
> She continued to be manic on the ward. She had been in this manic state for two or three months before being hospitalized. The very fact that she was brought to the hospital now and not several weeks before suggested that her behavior was becoming significantly more frantic and may have been signalling the end of the manic phase.
>
> Several weeks after she was hospitalized, she started complaining of intensified insomnia. Shortly thereafter she was severely depressed and had entered the depressive phase of her manic-depressive illness. The introduction of high doses of medication prevented severe insomnia from developing.
>
> This woman had been manic-depressive since her early 20s. Each year she experienced a shift of moods, spending some time feeling manic and energetic and some time feeling depressed. She cried often and was generally unable to sleep.

Pharmacological treatment that has been reasonably successful with this type of disorder is the administration of Lithium. This drug tends to stabilize mood shifts characteristic of mania and depression. All attendant symptoms, including insomnia, also tend to subside.

In addition to the relief brought by the correct medication, individuals with manic-depressive disorders are helped by psychotherapy to identify the symptoms preceding each major mood phase so that preventive measures may be taken to minimize their effect. Most of the time, people who are manic-depressive tend to deny the very obvious increase in their energy level as they enter the manic phase. Apparently, such individuals usually find it difficult to acknowledge the onset of these symptoms. As a matter of fact, most people who are depressed and who specifically develop the symptom of insomnia do not readily acknowledge psychological difficulties. Rather, they complain of their insomnia and, unfortunately, usually only seek medication to alleviate the symptom.

The entire clinical and diagnostic framework for insomnia can be divided into three parts. *First,* the prevailing behavior of the insomniac —the way such a person appears to others, as well as the way one experiences oneself—may reflect an ongoing and, in many cases, progressively deteriorating depression. *Second,* the emotions generated from this condition frequently include panic and irritability. Fundamentally, however, the emotion of anger plays a central role in the tendency for the depression to, so to speak, feed upon itself. A sense of loss or sorrow accompanies this anger and both the anger and sorrow are suppressed. This tendency for feelings to be suppressed then acts, in turn, to reinforce the depressive mood. One of the aims of any psychotherapeutic effort is to help depressed persons uncover and ventilate some of these suppressed feelings. *Third,* the underlying dependent structure of personality of many insomniacs contains an anxious hysterical quality during non-depressive times that covers an immovable, rigid and critical underlying paranoid stance. This kind of personality organization—behavior of depression, emotions of anger and sorrow and hysteric and paranoid elements—eventually produces many psychological, emotional and psychosomatic symptoms. One of the most prevalent of these symptoms is insomnia. Why insomnia should be a natural outgrowth of the blending of these personality characteristics will be considered in the following chapter.

Chapter 13

A Personality Analysis of Insomnia

INSOMNIA AND DECOMPENSATION

When insomnia becomes unbearable, it may be a signal that serious problems are brewing that are causing both the insomnia as well as a possible impending depressive or even decompensating process. This kind of phenomenon can even develop into a schizophrenic or psychotic process. All studies of sleep deprivation show that psychological, emotional and physical debilitation may occur in many conditions of severe insomnia and that, in some instances, the development of psychiatric conditions may also be observed (Hawkins, 1966, 1970; Mendels and Hawkins, 1971). General debilitation begins to occur at the prospect of lying in bed through the night, drifting in and out of sleep and feeling painfully alone. Frustration continues to mount at not getting that solid few hours of delicious, restful and peaceful sleep. Under such conditions, people begin to feel as if they have been cursed. The sufferer cannot explain it to anyone and is panicked about an increasingly fragmented life.

The six variations of depression with insomnia comprise a framework in which the vast majority of all conditions of insomnia may be understood. Only some of these conditions will eventually appear as part of a decompensating process. Others will simply continue to plague a person for many years in the absence of any major emotional fragmentation. In all of these conditions, a significant reduction of stage 4 delta sleep and/or REM sleep will be observed. If delta sleep is entirely eliminated, then a physical deterioration will surely occur. Furthermore, in such cases the insomnia may be so severe that it will reflect profound inner psychological and emotional turmoil and will raise the probability that REM sleep will also be eliminated. This is the condition frequently associated with decompensating processes, or at least seen in the development of psychiatric conditions (Agnew and Williams, 1964; Berger and Oswald, 1962; Hawkins et al., 1967; Kupfer, 1976; Sampson, 1966; Vogel, 1975; Williams, Ilaria and Karacan, 1979).

Interestingly enough, the disorder of schizophrenia and the appearance of insomnia are not usually found to be coexisting conditions (Bliss, 1967) except for the fact that in some chronic schizophrenic patients occasional mild sleep symptoms may be seen (Kupfer and Foster, 1975). If one is schizophrenic, then insomnia is likely not to be a symptom in one's overall repertoire of symptoms. A full discussion of sleep problems and schizophrenia is offered by Zarcone (1979). Insomnia does appear, however, in persons who are in the process of decompensating (Feinberg and Hiatt, 1978; Kupfer et al., 1970). Symptoms of decompensation include heightened anger or panic, a general reduction in concentration, and an overall irritability. After such a person has succumbed to the decompensating process and begun to express symptoms of schizophrenia such as delusions and hallucinations, insomnia tends to disappear.

During the process of decompensation, one most vividly experiences feelings of alienation. The decompensating person feels that too much is going on within to be able to explain or describe to anyone—even to one's closest friend or relative. To try to convey what is happening seems hopeless. It is this feeling of alienation that will generally appear in relation to the difficulty in the sequence and normal functioning of the stages of sleep.

In many studies of maladjustment, individuals experiencing decompensating feelings are shown to have greater levels of anger (Kellerman, 1965; Kellerman and Plutchik, 1968). Such anger is expressed in conjunction with an increasing sense that the world is chaotic, that there is nowhere to become anchored, and that one exists basically alone. The increased anger becomes most problematic at night. It creates an unusual sense of arousal and panic and keeps the person awake.

Yet, the typical dependent person with insomnia seems to have difficulty expressing anger. Like the narcoleptic, this person usually avoids confrontations, harbors the anger, and occasionally erupts at the wrong time and usually in an uncontrolled manner. Thus, an insomniac with this kind of problem is frequently in a high state of arousal. Bodily functions such as respiration, heartbeat and temperature are all increased. In addition, because of complaints of aches and pains and general malaise, such insomniacs are considered to be hypochondriacal; yet, they actually do seem to develop more psychosomatic problems than the normal sleeper.

The complaints of aches and pains and the appearance of actual psychosomatic symptoms in the insomniac can, at one time or another, include skin disorders, headache and other nervous or sensory problems, tightening in the chest, choking and other respiratory problems, all sorts of digestive disturbances such as heartburn, acidic stomach, and colitis, cardiovascular symptoms such as increased blood pressure, aches and pains in joints and muscles reflecting skeletomuscular problems, and sexual problems such as impotence. Insomniacs, therefore, especially those who are dependent and depressed, may begin to experience the process of the development of an entire catalogue of symptoms.

INSOMNIA, DEFENSES AND NIGHTMARES

The experience of heightened bodily symptoms, as well as the high state of arousal, also suggests that this kind of person may be lying awake because of a fear of dreaming. Prevailing theory suggests that, if one experiences intense psychological conflicts, a fear of sleeping may really represent a fear of dreaming. Since it is a prime assumption of psychoanalytic theory that one's inner conflicts are expressed in dreams, then usually the more intense these conflicts, the more the dreams they generate will reflect such intensity. Therefore, the insomniac is afraid to dream if an awake state can result.

There are various aspects of this theory that need to be amplified. Depending on one's psychological diagnosis and one's system of defense structure, the dreams of insomniacs, especially those who experience decompensating feelings, may be problematic because these dreams can turn into nightmares. This means that insomniacs may be afraid to sleep not simply because they are afraid to dream but more precisely because the fear of sleep is a fear of the appearance of nightmares. The question then becomes how does the system of defenses within one's personality operate to prevent nightmares as well as to release them?

THE MEANING OF NIGHTMARES

All dreams that awaken a person may be considered to be nightmares. Freud, in the very early part of the 20th century, examined in great detail the nature of the dream from his psychoanalytic point of view. He proposed that a successful dream is one that keeps the dreamer asleep. When inner conflicts are well disguised—the way dreams are thought to disguise them—the meaning of such conflicts is hidden and the dreamer, in the absence of feeling threatened, remains asleep. Conversely, when one's defenses cannot help disguise this kind of conflictual material, inner conflicts will not be hidden or disguised, threatening material will break into the dream in an undisguised way, and the dreamer will awaken with a nightmare.

Thus, all nightmares can produce mini-insomnia states—that is, states of heightened arousal during sleep time, interference with sleep, and, frequently, difficulty in getting back to sleep. These symptoms produced by nightmares resemble typical insomnia states: difficulty in falling asleep, wakefulness, and early morning premature rising. Yet, it is possible to experience nightmares and not suffer with insomnia. Furthermore, some insomniacs do not experience nightmares at all.

It has been proposed elsewhere (Kellerman, 1979, 1980) that

there are a small number of basic nightmare themes, not all of which are nightmares of terror. These nightmares emerge when a person's defenses are impaired to the extent that threatening material can no longer be managed. When this happens, significant changes in physical symptoms may occur. For example, the psychological defense of *displacement* is a central defense in the management of the emotion of anger. Displacement is defined as a mechanism of personality that can redirect anger. The classic example of displacement is exemplified by the individual who expresses his frustration at another person by kicking a chair. Kicking a chair is a displacement of the anger from the person toward whom it was originally intended to a less threatening object. In dreams, when anger and rage are intense and the mechanism of displacement is not sufficiently strong to manage such feelings or to redirect them, one may have a nightmare in which the dreamer becomes a menacing figure. To see oneself as a murderer or otherwise violent figure is usually unacceptable to the dreamer, and this sort of portrayal will generally produce a nightmare. It focuses too directly on the dreamer's anger and rage; to be so revealed becomes frequently threatening. In an opposite sense, when the mechanism of displacement is operating well, one's rage is well channeled or redirected and the dreamer can remain asleep dreaming some rather simple and innocuous dream.

Many insomniacs do not want to recognize their anger. Should such anger become extreme, nightmares may occur that force the dreamer to confront these angry feelings. It is only in this sense that insomniacs may be afraid to sleep—because to sleep is perchance to dream and perchance to have a nightmare. Furthermore, such nightmares are vivid and often remembered better than ordinary dreams. Remembering these angry or rageful kinds of nightmares makes any existing insomnia seem worse than it really is.

There are all sorts of dream-nightmare awakenings. For example, insomniacs who are sexually inhibited may experience blatant sexual dreams. Should such dreams be perceived as undesirable, they will awaken the dreamer. Dreams of terror are another example of nightmares that can awaken the dreamer. Still other nightmares include such sensations as loss of control, as in dreams of falling off buildings or mountains; paralysis, drowning or choking; grief, in which the dreamer awakens crying; and mutilation. These nightmares can occur when people, because of severe inner turmoil, no longer possess the defensive strength to deflect and disguise troublesome inner-conflict material.

The type of insomniac who is in a state of confusion, panic, and turmoil does not exercise sufficient self-control, so that nightmares of loss of control are possible. There are those who do not have the energy to defend against prohibited sexual feelings so that nightmares of sexuality may emerge. Furthermore, when one is highly frustrated and in a state of physiological arousal, the defense mechanism of displacement cannot adequately rechannel extra anger and, therefore, nightmares of rage may occur. When one's positive self-image is undermined, it may not be possible to utilize the defense mechanism of compensation. As a result, feelings of loss and separation, akin to those that are experienced when a death has occurred, may generate nightmares of grief. Other nightmares can include themes of fragmentation in which one's body literally falls apart. Such nightmares may occur when the defense mechanism of projection is impaired. Projection is the mechanism that allows people to avoid seeing their own faults by noticing similar faults in others. Thus, without the projection defense mechanism, people who are always critical of others would tend to criticize themselves. The body fragmentation nightmare reflects the ultimate self-criticism. Such nightmares occur in critical-paranoid people whose projected criticality is blocked. There may also be nightmares of sensory experiences that include hypnagogic, hallucinatory-like states.

All these formulations indicate that, in debilitating conditions such as insomnia, the entire defense structure of personality is worn thin. As a result, the insomniac will be in a most vulnerable position with respect to the appearance of nightmares. The elimination of REM-dream periods during severe attacks of insomnia therefore creates a paradox. On the one hand, an absence of dreams may in fact provide the insomniac with relief from the debilitating effects of potential frequent nightmares. On the other hand, an absence of dreams can produce greater tension in the personality. Nightmares will ultimately be associated with insomnia, however, because of the damage to the defense system of personality that occurs in prolonged conditions of insomnia.

THE USE OF FANTASY TO TREAT INSOMNIA

The use of pleasant fantasies or daydreams can have some ameliorative effect on the condition of insomnia. Persons with insomnia have reported that thinking of a specific fantasy has helped them calm down and ultimately fall asleep.

> A man, 33 years of age, who was experiencing moderate insomnia both with respect to falling asleep and in terms of wakefulness after falling asleep, happened to hit upon a fantasy that enabled him to drift off into sleep. He would imagine that a certain friend of his died and that this friend's wife needed to be consoled. The upshot was that they started a relationship that was warm and loving.
>
> This patient had been harboring a secret crush on his friend's wife but was careful never to reveal his feelings either in words or in deeds. He was obsessed by this woman's large breasts, and thinking about possessing her was the key to his newfound tranquility. This fantasy also contains the psychological ingredients found in the onset of insomnia and in its ultimate resolution. The fantasy of the friend's death reflects *separation* concerns, while the creation of a relationship with his wife reflects the possibility of satisfying dependency needs.

Fantasies of sex, of heroic deeds, or of any other compensatory act may sometimes help insomnia sufferers to sleep. This means that whatever fantasy can be applied to elevate one's self-image may help reduce the tensions causing the sleep problem. The point is that the fantasy must be of a compensatory nature—something that makes one feel good, strong, happy, vindicated, powerful, influential, recognized, applauded, adored, admired, feared, needed, protected, etc. In some cases relief from anxiety may also be achieved by fantasizing acts of supplication or submission. Sooner or later the insomnia sufferer may hit upon either the particular compensatory or guilt-alleviating theme that will help.

Patients have also reported that masturbation can alleviate the tension of insomnia. Some people indeed report being able to fall asleep only by masturbating while others report that masturbating generates greater tension, thereby making it more difficult to sleep. It should be remembered, nevertheless, that fantasy, if used successfully, can sometimes have a profound effect on mood changes.

CAN THE DAY'S EVENTS CAUSE INSOMNIA?

A day's event in itself can cause insomnia only if some part of the event contained a special symbolic or psychological meaning for the person. Freud (1900), in his discussion of how the day's events influence dreams, originally proposed this idea. He indicated that not all events of the day are psychologically salient for the person. What happens, presumably, is that the individual is constantly scanning and evaluating all of the day's events in an unconscious automatic manner as they occur. Those events that in some special way represent something currently important or evoke feelings that are reminiscent of important past experiences will probably be retained and then appear in some manner in the dream.

It would seem that the same principle could apply to the influence of the day's events on the difficult sleep of the insomniac. When a person suffering from insomnia is asked to describe the day's events, not all events are described, nor are they necessarily listed in precise chronological sequence; they may be distorted to some extent, and sometimes they can be entirely forgotten. The point is that because of each person's special needs and typical defensive patterns, and because not all of the day's events are of equal significance, only some events have the capacity to affect one's sleep. Such events, if they possess symbolic significance, may contribute to the reinforcement of already existing insomnia. This significance will frequently refer to issues of *dependency, separation, and the general condition of one's important relationships*.

A DIAGNOSTIC CASE ILLUSTRATION

A woman of 40 who was admitted to a state hospital for a severe depressive phase of a manic-depressive episode, was evaluated with psychological tests. These tests included the standard battery of projective tests: the Rorschach inkblot test, the Thematic Apperception Test (TAT) and the Human Figure Drawing Analysis Test. The Emotions Profile Index (EPI)—a test that measures how people rate themselves in terms of emotions and personality traits was also included.

The patient had been hospitalized in previous years for similar episodes of depression. She would usually become depressed and would stop sleeping. After not sleeping for several weeks, she would become incoherent.

Results on the psychological tests showed that this woman was an exceptionally dependent person whose expectations of relationships resembled those more typical of children. She was an action-oriented person, quite immature and completely non-introspective. She expected that all of her needs would be taken care of but did not ever wonder how she might help herself. She was usually a moody person and results showed that her mood swings could be expected to recur.

On the Rorschach inkblot test she was quite scattered and severely constrained by her depression. Her stories on the TAT and her drawings revealed that she was not a terribly well-controlled person and that she was quite capable of "spilling over." Thus, she could be impulsive and she had poor tolerance for frustration. Generally she did not have the emotional resources to cope with undue stress.

The Emotions Profile Index (Plutchik and Kellerman, 1974) was administered when she was depressed, again two months later when her depression lifted, and a third time several months later when, as an outpatient at the hospital, she developed an acute manic state.

Results are quite interesting. During all three phases, the depressed, the more stable and the manic, her distrustfulness score—a score that implies paranoid dissatisfaction and criticality—remained relatively high despite the changes in all other scores.

Figure 13.1 shows EPI profiles during each of her three phases: when she was manic, depressed, and reasonably stable.

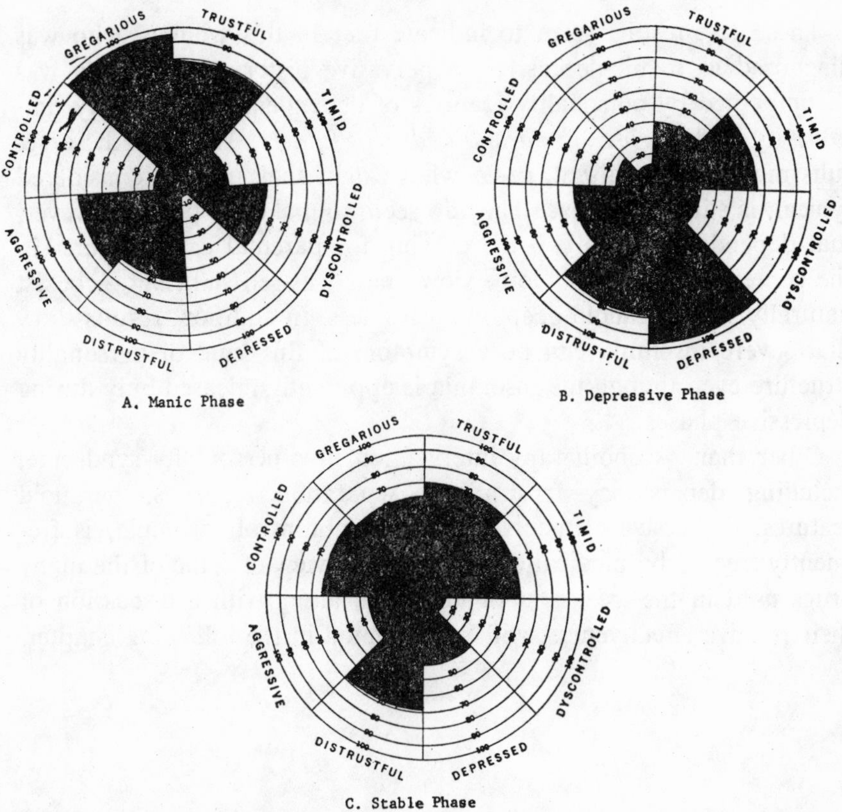

FIGURE 13.1: Emotion Profile Index scores of a 40-year-old hospitalized female manic-depressive patient with severe insomnia. A. During manic phase; B. During depressive phase; and, C. During reasonably stable phase. The center of the circle represents zero percent and the outer ring of the circle represents 100 percent.

When she was depressed her sociability score was low, depression score was high and paranoid score was high. When she was stable her depression score was much lower, her sociability score much higher and yet her distrustful-paranoid score remained relatively high.

Finally, when she was in the manic state, depression was absent, her sociability score was very high and her distrustfulness score only slightly lowered.

These test results seem to indicate that in this woman, who was diagnosed as manic-depressive, a pervasive history of insomnia was accompanied by personality features of dependency, immaturity, impulsivity and *a core of paranoid distrustfulness.* Whether these results may be generalized, or to what extent they may be considered typical, is still speculative. They do seem to make the point, however, that dependency features—the craving for parental caring figures in the context of being unable to view oneself as self-sufficient—coexist naturally with paranoid deep distrustfulness. In addition, results show that severe insomnia can be a symptom of this kind of personality structure even though the insomnia is apparently released only during depressive phases.

Other than psychotherapy intervention, this personality syndrome, including dependency frustrations, separation anxieties, paranoid features, depressive elements and the symptom of insomnia, is frequently treated by medication. A general review of some of the many drugs used in the treatment of insomnia, along with a discussion of their relative effectiveness, will be presented in the following chapter.

Chapter 14

The Use of Medication in the Treatment of Insomnia

DISTURBANCE OF BRAIN ACTIVITY IN INSOMNIA

It has been suggested in the scientific literature that insomnia may be caused by a disturbance of the arousal system or of the inhibitory sleep system of the brain (Hartmann, 1976; Magoun, 1952, 1958). What this means is that insomnia—as an example of a sleep disorder—results from an injury or incapacity of the body's normal mechanisms of sleep to check or inhibit its waking system. This point was reviewed in Chapter 5.

The waking system, located in the reticular formation of the brain (Akert, 1965), is typically bombarded by cortical electrical stimulation. In order for a person to sleep, this excitement of the waking system needs to be inhibited (Moruzzi and Magoun, 1949; Netter, 1968). In a sense, the waking system needs to be put to sleep in order for actual sleep to take place. The problem in the correct or incorrect inhibiting of the waking system can be seen, then, to involve possible neurological, physiological, chemical and psychological effects. In people who experience anxiety states—that is, conditions of great psychic tension and inner turmoil—the waking system may be excessively stimulated so that insomnia is a natural effect of this anxiety.

The entire arousal system needs to become more dormant if insomnia is to subside and if the probability of sleep is to increase. The inhibition of the arousal or waking system occurs by the ever-decreasing contact with the external world. What this means is that more and more distance from the external world is achieved by the gradual inhibition of function of the muscles, skin and sense organs—especially those of seeing and hearing. Some authors believe that the disappearance of much of stage 4 delta sleep in the aged may be a result of injury or loss of cortical cells due to age and manifested by a decrease in function of the inhibitory system. This would explain the typical insomnia seen in the aged. Furthermore, any lesions or injury to various parts of the reticular formation of the brain can also lead to a decrease of REM-dream stages. This condition of the brain can also explain the pre-psychotic experience or the process of decompensation of people who miss a consistent amount of delta stage 4 sleep or REM-dream sleep.

For the most part, the use of drugs in the treatment of insomnia plays an important part in influencing the functions of the reticular formation of the brain. The main objective in the use of some of this medication is to help in the inhibition of the reticular activating system or the awake system of the brain so that an increase in the probability of sleep may occur.

In the following section, the nature of this medication, its physical and psychological effects on the insomniac, and the way in which such medications affect those brain functions that are most responsible for the regulation of sleepfulness and wakefulness will be presented.

SLEEP MEDICATION

There are many sleep medications generally known as hypnotic sedatives that have been used in the treatment of insomnia (Cooper, 1977; Kales, Bixler, Tan et al., 1974; Kales et al., 1969). The variety of drugs that are used certainly implies that a standard drug treatment for insomnia has not yet been firmly established (Kales and Kales, 1970; Kales et al., 1977; Oswald, 1968). These drugs may be divided into two categories—the barbiturates and the non-barbiturates. Among the barbiturates—those that are addictive—are Amytal,

Seconal, Nembutal, and Luminal. Among the non-barbiturates—those that are presumably non-addictive—are the drugs called *benzodiazepines* such as Dalmane, Valium, Tranxene, Serax, Librium, and the popular drug called Miltown—a *propanediol.* In addition, the antidepressant drugs, Elavil and Sinequan, are commonly used in the treatment of insomnia.

A further introduction to psychopharmacology is offered in Ban (1969), Holliday (1965), Honigfeld (1973), and Rech and Moore (1971). Additional studies of the effect of sedative hypnotic drugs are reviewed in Cooper (1977), Kales et al. (1977), Kales, Bixler, Tan et al. (1974), and Ware (1979). Oswald (1969) also discusses sleep and dependence on drugs. The tricyclic antidepressant drugs are discussed by Klerman and Paykel (1970), and Malitz (1966). The barbiturates, non-barbiturates, benzodiazepines, propanediols, and tricyclic antidepressants are reported in considerable detail in the annual Physicians' Desk Reference with respect to dosage and possible side effects of the various medications. These will be outlined in the following sections.

Barbiturates

Barbiturates are addictive. People who use such drugs have a tendency to want to increase their dosages as time passes. This can be quite dangerous because overdoses can be fatal. These drugs have side effects that should be noted. With increased dosages they can cause abdominal discomfort, such as nausea; they can also cause skin rashes, mental confusion, dizziness, and the feeling of hangover. They tend to decrease REM-dreaming, which in certain cases may actually aggravate conditions of insomnia (Oswald et al., 1963). If they do, in fact, produce a decrease or inhibition in REM-dreaming, then other side effects will occur such as agitation, anxiety, and even additional and more visible depression.

One of the theories of the positive functions of the barbiturates is that they will depress cortical activity—that is, they will depress the activity from the cortex that stimulates the reticular activating system or the wakeful system of the brain. When activity from the cortex is decreased, then the wakeful reticular activating system will become gradually deactivated and ultimately it will become inhibited. This inhibiting process permits the function of those systems in the brain that generate sleep. Eventually, with such inhibition, the troubled sleeper will sleep.

Short Acting Barbiturates—Amytal (*sodium amobarbital*) is a rapid-acting barbiturate commonly used for the relief of anxiety. It is prescribed for people who are having difficulty falling asleep. It is a sedative and a hypnotic drug. Some negative side effects can include hangover and pain. For insomnia, 65-200 milligrams are recommended by mouth at bedtime. The effect of the drug may be experienced in less than one half hour.

Seconal (*secobarbital sodium*) is a drug also used for sedation. It is frequently prescribed for the treatment of insomnia and is a short-acting sedative and hypnotic. Its effect is prompt. It can cause negative side effects in the form of hangover and pain. The usual dosage recommended is 100 milligrams at bedtime. Overdosages can be fatal, especially if associated with alcohol abuse. It can also cause mild anesthesia and drowsiness.

Intermediate Acting Barbiturates—Nembutal (*phenobarbital elixir*) is a short-to-intermediate-acting barbiturate commonly used for insomnia and anxiety. It acts as a sedative and hypnotic. Its effect is rapid and will be experienced in about 30 minutes. Its action ranges from three to six hours. Potential negative side effects may include rash, allergic reactions, severe depression, drowsiness, hangover and nausea. The usual hypnotic dose given is 100 milligrams.

Long Acting Barbiturate—Luminal (*sodium phenobarbital*) is used as a sedative. It is also sometimes used as a hypnotic to replace Scopolamine—sometimes referred to as the *truth serum*. It is reported to be effective in the treatment of depression, agitation, anxiety and insomnia. The usual dosage prescribed for this drug ranges between 100 and 300 milligrams. Luminal may have some of the same negative side effects reported for all other barbiturates.

Non-Barbiturates

The non-barbiturate drugs, although presumably not addictive, may nevertheless have certain addictive effects with high dosages. They may also generate many negative side effects, including the feeling of dependence or psychological addiction. They may be divided into three broad categories: the benzodiazepines, which are non-lethal but may become dangerous if mixed with alcohol; the propanediols, that may have toxic reactions similar to those of barbiturates; and the tricyclic antidepressant drugs.

Benzodiazepines

Drugs within the category benzodiazepines are generally non-lethal unless taken by people who are also prone to the use of alcohol. These drugs are used for the treatment of anxiety. They have a long duration of action.

Dalmane (*flurazepam hydrochloride*) has been reported to produce the best results for insomnia, in certain respects, because it can be taken for approximately 28 consecutive nights. It is an hypnotic agent prescribed for symptoms of insomnia, including difficulty in falling asleep, frequent nocturnal awakenings, and early morning awakenings. It is taken at bedtime in doses ranging from 15 to 30 milligrams. Adverse reactions may include dizziness and drowsiness. Overdosage also can produce nausea, nervousness, constipation, and coma. Results indicate that the best effects of this drug with respect to the relief of insomnia require three or four nights of continuous use.

Valium (*diazepam*) is used for the relief of tension, anxiety, fatigue, depressive symptoms, and agitation. After prolonged use, if Valium is abruptly discontinued, some withdrawal symptoms may appear. Some negative side effects can include dizziness, drowsiness, and drunken-like gait. Some paradoxical excitement such as hyperexcited states, hallucinations, and insomnia have been reported. In adults, 5-20 milligrams daily is usually prescribed.

Tranxene (*clorazepate dipotassium*) is taken for the relief of anxiety, usually in patients over 18 years of age. It may also cause some withdrawal symptoms after abrupt discontinuance. These withdrawal symptoms include insomnia, irritability and diarrhea. The main side effect of this drug is drowsiness. Other side effects can include gastrointestinal complaints, blurred vision, dry mouth, and even mental confusion. Still other side effects can include insomnia, rashes, slurred speech, irritability and depression. The usual daily dosage of this drug is 7.5-30 milligrams. A 15-milligram single dose at bedtime is recommended.

Serax (*oxazepam*) is used to control anxiety, tension, agitation, and anxiety associated with depression. Adverse reactions have been few but have included mild drowsiness, dizziness, vertigo and headache. Some mild paradoxical reactions such as stimulation of affect have also been reported. More infrequent side effects can include rashes, nausea, lethargy, tremor, and slurred speech. Dosages recommended range from 15 to 60 milligrams daily.

Librium (*chlordiazepoxide hydrochloride*) is a drug used for the relief of anxiety and tension. Overdoses have resulted in confusion, coma and diminished reflexes. Otherwise, negative side effects that are infrequently reported include drowsiness, skin eruptions, minor menstrual irregularities, changes in one's sexual drive, and nausea and constipation. In adults, 10-50 milligrams daily is the recommended dosage.

Propanediols

Drugs within the category propanediols can be toxic. These drugs can generate significant physical dependence and they have a shorter duration of clinical benefit. The most popular and frequently used propanediol is Miltown.

Miltown (*meprobamate*) is prescribed for the relief of anxiety and tension. It is also used specifically to promote sleep in tense patients. Side effects have included slurred speech, physical and psychological dependence, and vertigo. Sudden discontinuance can cause insomnia, anorexia, and various withdrawal reactions such as tremors, vomiting, confusion, rash, headaches, and severe depression. Dosages for adults can be applied in amounts of 200-600 milligrams daily, or up to 1,600 milligrams divided into three or four doses daily.

Tricyclic Antidepressants with Sedative Effect

In the use of tricyclic antidepressant drugs such as Elavil, Tofranil and Sinequan, the antidepressant effects usually take up to two weeks to appear in most severe depressions. These drugs can be dangerous if taken in overdose. They are particularly dangerous to cardiac patients.

Elavil (*amitriptyline hydrochloride*) is an antidepressant sedative. It works best for persons suffering with depression accompanied by anxiety. Dosage recommendation ranges between 10-75 milligrams per day. In some cases it can take up to one month for the effects of the drug to develop. Negative side effects can include confusional states, excitement, insomnia, tremors, skin rash, nausea, peculiar taste, changed (usually lowered) levels of sexual drive, testicular swelling, breast enlargement, drowsiness and headache.

Sinequan (*doxepin hydrochloride*) is recommended for persons who experience anxiety and depression. It works well for symptoms of general tension, anxiety, depression, lack of energy, and sleep disturbance. It is relatively safe but is not recommended for children under 12. It should also be ruled out for patients with glaucoma. Adverse reactions may include dry mouth, blurred vision, drowsiness, rash, nausea and vomiting, changes in sexual drive, weight gain, headache and fatigue. The usual recommended dosage may range between a low of 25-50 milligrams and a high of 75-150 milligrams per day.

Tofranil (*imipramine hydrochloride*) is used for the relief of depression—usually those that are of long duration. The usual dosage recommended ranges between 50-100 milligrams daily. Adverse reactions may include palpitation, confusion, anxiety, insomnia, tremors, dry mouth, blurred vision, rash, nausea, change in sexual drive, weight gain or loss and headache.

Both the barbiturates and non-barbiturates have the reputation of becoming ineffective in long-term treatment use. Yet for short-term relief required by people who cannot sleep, they frequently can be very helpful. People who use these drugs, however, tend to increase their dosages because, as one becomes accustomed to a standard dose, its effect may not be as powerful as it was originally. Another problem is the physiological effect of some of the short-acting hypnotic drugs which can and do produce nightmares.

The main effects of the barbiturates are their sedation and sleep-induction qualities. Since tolerance to them develops rapidly, there is an ever-present danger of abuse (Oswald and Priest, 1965). The benzodiazepines also contain sedative, hypnotic and anti-convulsive properties; however, they also possess the remarkable ability to reduce anxiety and aggression. These also have become common drugs for abuse. Although they can become habit-forming, the actual occurrence of physiological dependence is low. With Librium and Valium, any serious withdrawal reactions would emerge five to seven days after the discontinuance of medication.

The antidepressants are frequently quite effective in relieving insomnia. Zung (1970) indicates that they "stimulate the limbic system—a physiological center for emotion—and therefore they will improve one's mood." Furthermore, they "stimulate the hypothalamus and therefore improve the various biological dysfunctions present in depression such as decreased appetite, sleep and libido" or sexual functioning. Third, they "inhibit the reticular formation which further improves the sleep disturbance." Fourth, they "increase the neurohumoral depots, which are deficient in depressive disorders."

In addition, antidepressants such as Tofranil and Elavil will decrease the number of awakenings of the insomniac. These drugs will increase stage 4 delta sleep—the all-important deepest, most relaxed and restorative sleep. They will also, unfortunately, decrease REM-dreaming and finally, they will increase the duration of the normal 90-minute sleep-dream cycle (Zung, 1968).

Elavil can also alleviate tensions sufficiently so that more hostility can emerge in dreams. This is important because the appearance of hostility in dreams can reflect a lessening of rigidity, an overall process of getting better, and a decrease in general agitation. The appearance of hostility in dreams also frequently corresponds to better and more peaceful overall sleep. Pervasive rage in dreams, however, can signal a decompensating process.

The antidepressants such as Elavil, Sinequan and Tofranil even help those people to sleep better who do not actually feel depressed, but who nevertheless experience insomnia. Valium, not technically an antidepressant, is also used frequently to help people sleep. However, individuals who use Valium are generally those who are tense and anxious. Valium is a drug that can cause withdrawal symptoms, while Elavil, Sinequan and Tofranil generally do not. Withdrawal is a serious problem especially in the use of barbiturates (Kales et al., 1968) and in the use of some hypnotic drugs that tend to decrease stage 4 delta sleep. They can also cause suicidal feelings in severe chronic insomnia patients.

Most medication for insomnia, especially if used over a long period of time, may eventually be ineffective. From time to time, symptoms of insomnia also paradoxically appear. There are, however, many individuals who have been using antidepressants or other medication for depression and insomnia for many years with good results. Many of the people who use sleep medication need the psychological reassurance it provides in order to feel secure. This is an area of research that needs to be further studied. It is essentially the study of the pharmacology of sleep (Kay et al., 1976) as it interacts with psychological problems of individuals.

RESISTANCE TO PSYCHOTHERAPY

Many people with insomnia resist recognizing their own psychological conflicts and problems. Physicians frequently propose to their insomnia patients that they may be in need of psychological or psychiatric consultation only to be summarily disregarded. Usually, such persons are interested only in symptom relief. They want to sleep, not to talk about the things that bother them. They frequently are not sure precisely what is bothering them—as in cases of people with free-floating anxieties—or they are not consciously feeling disturbed at all, except for the inability to sleep.

Because the typical insomnia sufferer has been reported to be resistive to psychological treatment, it is implied that insomnia may be the kind of symptom developed by individuals who are not introspective types—those who tend not to want to look within in order to examine their conflicts. Nonintrospective individuals are those who typically do not ask themselves why they feel depressed and anxious.

> A woman in her 80s with a lifelong history of insomnia starting at the age of 20 was troubled with her insomnia only until she married at the age of 26. After she was married, her condition continued unabated but it did not disturb her.
>
> This woman had been sleeping only four hours per night for the past 60 years. She had the most interesting hobbies and would spend her time in the small hours of the morning sewing, knitting, reading and working on some project. She felt blissful throughout this wakefulness and would steal little catnaps during the day.
>
> She was so content with her marriage generally and with her husband specifically that his mere presence—even though he was sleeping—permitted her to feel comfortable with her insomnia.
>
> She was admitted to the hospital one week after her husband died at 92. He was not ill preceding his death; she discovered him expired in bed in the morning. He had died uneventfully in his sleep. She had no time to prepare emotionally for his death and she became depressed, disoriented, and suddenly terribly frantic about her inability to sleep.
>
> She was visited on the hospital ward by a psychiatric resident who, in taking her history, asked her about her lifelong condition of insomnia, when and why it started, how she managed it, and so forth. It appeared, not so surprisingly, that she was virtually unaware of any of these details with respect to the development of her insomnia.

The fact that this woman was so unaware of, or even unconcerned with, her condition is an extreme example of the reason many insomniacs never seek help. Such persons just do not realize or perhaps do not want to know that insomnia can be a symptom of some latent emotional problem. The unfortunate side effect of this lack of awareness or of this defensive posture is that often insomnia can be quickly traced and its origin can be pinpointed. However, because of a lack of awareness individuals will not seek help to resolve whatever latent conflicts exist. Through psychotherapy consultation and in a relatively short period of time, the insomnia symptom can be eliminated. Of course, the value of such consultation is that it can be useful in the working-through of inner conflicts such as depression and other debilitating states.

Whereas narcolepsy needs to be treated with drugs, insomnia can quite often, even in the majority of cases, be treated entirely with psychotherapy. Yet, insomnia frequently has to be episodic to the point of suicidal depression before psychotherapy will be considered. In the long run, insomnia can be reinforced instead of abated by the use of drugs, especially when the insomnia is not acutely severe. The insomniac who opts for drugs instead of psychotherapy treatment may be really creating conditions for the reinforcement of the insomnia.

The trade-off that people are willing to make for short-term relief is understandable. Yet, the prospect of reinforcing insomnia by creating a drug dependence or by creating for oneself a false sense of security is not terribly wise and in many cases it is actually senseless. In fact, Ware (1979) states, "A common misconception has been that hypnotic medications restore normal sleep. To the contrary, hypnotic medications distort normal sleep when used appropriately and destroy all normal sleep when misused." Furthermore, Kales, Bixler, Tan et al. (1974) warn that insomnia can even be induced by the abrupt withdrawal of hypnotic drugs.

Psychotherapy is a treatment that can reveal underlying causes for insomnia and depression. This sometimes occurs when the patient's experiences become analyzed with respect to *dependency issues* and *issues of separation*. In therapy, these issues are examined, analyzed and transformed so that the conflicts such symptoms represent may be resolved. When one chooses drugs instead of psychotherapy, long-range improvement may be minimal. Psychotherapy should be the treatment of choice by insomniacs, whether or not they rely on medication.

Although medication for insomnia may be necessary, many insomniacs use such drugs to resist psychological consultation. They may be apprehensive or embarrassed about becoming identified as a patient in therapy. They also may be fearful of examining what is perhaps felt to be the terrible secrets that many people think they harbor. Their decision is to let sleeping tigers sleep. If this be the case, such reasons have no basis in reality. In contemporary society, many people are in therapy or seeking therapy. Second, the deep recesses or secrets of one's mind are not necessarily bad or to be avoided. These recesses can be interesting and quite illuminating. Because of such biases, however, insomniacs may unnecessarily suffer for their entire lives with this disorder. Many psychoanalysts would probably agree that such individuals may need to retain the insomnia symptom because it qualifies as something to complain about—a secondary gain symptom. If one were to ask persons with insomnia whether they need to retain the symptom, such a suggestion probably would be vehemently denied. This is unfortunate because in the vast majority of cases insomnia can be completely eliminated through psychotherapy. When psychotherapy is avoided, the sleeping tiger may sleep, but the insomniac doesn't.

Part IV

THEORY AND SYNTHESIS

Chapter 15

Insomnia and Narcolepsy: A Synthesis

THE NEED FOR DEPENDENCY AND ITS RELATION TO INSOMNIA AND NARCOLEPSY

In this book an attempt has been made to describe the causes, the symptoms and the potential control of both insomnia and narcolepsy. It has been indicated that these disorders share common themes but reflect very different poles of these themes.

It has also been proposed in earlier chapters that disappointment in the satisfaction of dependency needs is likely to generate sleep problems during times of separation from an important relationship. This need for dependence is developed at an early time in one's life; it essentially means the search for togetherness or *attachment* (Parens and Saul, 1971).

The connection between the process of attachment and the development of dependency needs has also been described by Bowlby (1973). Bowlby indicates that people who experience intense dependency needs are those who, during infancy and childhood, experienced a difficult attachment process with parents or parental surrogates. The effect of difficult early attachment experiences can produce problems centering around whether or not to really trust others or, rather, to be suspicious and distrust them. Bowlby points out that early attachment problems are extremely powerful. They can continue into and pervade adult life. Individuals who have difficult attachment problems may always feel that they will never be comfortable unless they can carefully control all relationships. Dependency needs and subsequent attachment problems examined with respect to insomnia and narcolepsy are viewed in the discussions throughout this book basically in terms of such object relations concerns. This issue of attachment has also been discussed in the psychoanalytic literature in terms of symbiotic relationships and the process of individuation (Bergman, 1971; Mahler, 1968), and the field of object relations theory is essentially one concerned with early relationships and their effects on development (Jacobson, 1964; Kernberg, 1977; Kohut, 1977; Schafer, 1968; Winnicott, 1953). In fact, all psychoanalytic theories recognize the importance of object relations and its role in the appearance of dependency as well as attachment problems (Freud, 1923; Guntrip, 1968; Mahler et al., 1975).

Dependency and attachment experiences are ultimately connected to emotions and personality. The emotions most involved seem to be related to attitudes of trustfulness and distrustfulness. Basically, this means that if one has experienced reasonable satisfaction in early attachment events, then that person can be more trusting of relationships in the present. However, if attachment experiences have been problematic, then frequent doubting of relationships and never fully trusting them are likely to develop. The deeper meaning of dependency, then, may be associated with opposite elements of personality that can be identified as traits of trustfulness and distrustfulness.

These opposite emotions of trust and distrust seem to revolve around the need to form attachments and achieve satisfactions by depending on a partner, but they also create a dilemma with respect to how one conducts any relationship. The dilemma may be posed simply as, "Do I trust my partner or don't I?" The dependent and passive narcoleptic person may answer, "I would like to, but underneath I'm afraid to be rejected." On the other hand, the dependent person with insomnia may respond to this imaginary dilemma by saying, "Yes, I do trust, but I am basically not convinced that it is a good idea." The narcoleptic person may be somewhat guarded on top and susceptible underneath, while the person with insomnia is apparently accepting and trusting above but fundamentally suspicious and skeptical underneath. Many dependent people who either are narcoleptic or have insomnia constantly struggle with these opposite inclinations towards others—of trustful and distrustful orientations—but they experience their respective problems in different ways.

The inclination to be trusting or distrusting has specific relations to one's personality and psychological diagnosis. In psychological and psychiatric language, an overtrusting person is also frequently optimistic, impetuous and highly suggestible, and is usually defined as an energized hysterical type. A distrustful person is frequently described as suspicious, rigid, skeptical and guarded and is usually defined as a critical paranoid type. Thus, theoretically many dependent narcoleptic persons, whether depressed, compulsive or passive, may be more basically distrustful and somewhat paranoid on top, and overtrustful or hysterical beneath the surface; that is, such a person can appear to be immovable but may actually be suggestible. In contrast, many dependent persons with insomnia, whether depressed, compulsive, manic, or passive, may more basically be trustful, suggestible and hysteric on the surface but remain distrustful, intractable, somewhat paranoid, suspicious, and rigid underneath. Such a person may appear to be suggestible and cooperative but may actually be quite immovable. Thus, the dependent narcoleptic person is distrustful above and overtrustful beneath the surface, while the dependent person with insomnia is trustful above but distrustful underneath.

The psychological aspect to the sleep attack experienced by the dependent narcoleptic person relates in part to the inability to bear the sense that at any given moment one can be deeply subject to suggestion and influence. There is a sense of a lack of solidity—that no matter what the conviction is regarding any decision or opinion, it is vulnerable to the persuasion of others. This fear reveals the narcoleptic person's underlying susceptibility that is perhaps based upon an everpresent trustful hope for attachment and dependency. The dependent person with insomnia, on the other hand, seems to be "all ears" on the surface. Whatever suggestions are made by doctors, friends or relatives are eagerly received and seemingly accepted with great appreciation. Yet, before long, and even before such plans are implemented, modifications are made, medication is manipulated, and finally plans become discarded. Thus, this sort of person appears to be trusting on the surface but basically doubts all commitments and hardly shows any capacity to be influenced beneath a surface of receptivity.

What is it in the personality structures and in the respective histories of dependent persons with narcolepsy and insomnia that produce such similar personality themes and yet such distinctly opposite personalities and correspondingly distinctly opposite sleep problems? The answer to this question lies in the nature of early family experiences—until adolescence—with respect to parent-child relationships. Sleep problems relate to how the attachment process was experienced and whether dependency needs were met in appropriate ways. The connections between dependency needs, attachment processes, fears of separation, depression, hysterical-trustfulness, paranoid-distrustfulness, and the emotions of anger and fear are all-important to the understanding of the onset of narcolepsy and insomnia, especially in such dependent persons.

WHAT DOES "DEPENDENCY" MEAN FOR PERSONS WITH NARCOLEPSY OR INSOMNIA?

The nature of early family relationships provides one framework for understanding how dependency needs developed (Bowlby, 1973; Mahler, 1968). All people need to be cared for and to feel secure in the knowledge that parents or parental figures will be attentive, loving and instructive. Children depend on their parents, but also expect that their parents will help them grow up in a way that enables them to take care of themselves. They want their parents to do things for them—but not all things. When parents do help, are loving and do indeed encourage an appropriate amount of independent action, then children are able to experience their attachments in a healthy manner and do not feel angry because they think too much is being done for them or that hardly anything at all is being done for them.

Neurotic dependency, therefore, may be avoided if children are not unnecessarily infantilized, on the one hand, nor ignored but expected coldly to perform on the other. This is an important point because at each stage of infancy and childhood one has to master certain tasks and expectations in order to traverse these "passages" successfully (Erikson, 1963; Kohut, 1977; Winnicott, 1953). Attachment processes and dependency needs become problematic when the child is either overcontrolled and infantilized or to a great extent ignored. In such cases, both the overcontrolled child and the one who is ignored yearn for more appropriate attachments. Either experience may result in intense dependency needs in later years. These inordinate needs can produce problems in relationships because people will express them, in part, to control these relationships. For example, individuals who were overcontrolled may need to monitor relationships closely because of the profound inferiority feelings that resulted from these early experiences and because they are always so afraid of losing the adored partner. Such persons so desperately need to depend on others that they can become frightened by these very needs. A typical defensive or coping response to this fear is to appear blasé, independent, or even defiant. Others, who have been deprived of a significant amount and healthy kind of attachment, can appear, on the surface, to welcome relationships but underneath may basically distrust them. Such individuals may essentially remain detached even though they may currently need and may have always needed close relationships. In either case, the problem sleeper is likely to be poorly differentiated from parental figures. What this means is that overdependent people who were not permitted enough independent action do not really know where they begin and their parents end (Jacobson, 1964; Kernberg, 1977). Persons who were expected to be superindependent but were deprived of sufficient nurturance can crave dependent attachment because it had never been originally achieved in any satisfying way.

An example of the effect of infantilized development on mood is the experience of new mothers who develop postpartum depression. Physicians are likely to attribute the appearance of this kind of depression to chemical and hormonal changes, but such explanations are not always made with much conviction. What, then, can be another explanation for this kind of depression? Perhaps the answer can be found in the mother's perception and feeling about a new person in her life and the impact that this new relationship implies. An index of the mother's own maturity level can signal whether or not a postpartum depression will occur at all. If the new mother feels able to meet the demands of this dependent infant, then the probability of any kind of depression is surely decreased. If, on the other hand, the mother suddenly begins to feel that such demands will be too much for her to manage or that her identity has shifted for the worse—meaning she must be mature—then depression can develop along with a variety of other symptoms. One of these symptoms can be insomnia.

> Rachel, a 36-year-old woman, was pregnant with her second child. During her first pregnancy several years before, she would periodically become upset at seemingly unimportant circumstances. Yet, after the birth of this first child, she was able to manage his needs and was not at all depressed.
>
> She was a very dependent person, and in her formative years was never required to meet even the most conventional demands. She was not required to work, shop, tidy up her room, and so forth. These things were always done for her. Furthermore, her homework became quite a chore for her and she eventually stopped doing all assignments. She was quite indulged throughout her life and was, more or less, preoccupied only with her social life. Her unlimited and inappropriate use of credit cards in her adult years essentially defined the principles of her life—"buy now and let the future take care of itself." As an adult, Rachel remained a spoiled child. She was unprepared to care for herself in a mature way. Nevertheless, with her husband's help she seemed to be able to manage some of the needs of her new family.
>
> During her second pregnancy, she developed symptoms of anxiety. Thereafter she experienced a serious post-partum de-

pression after the birth of this child. One of her symptoms was a sleeping disturbance. As it first appeared, she tended to oversleep. After some weeks she found she could not sleep at all, felt very dissatisfied, and dreaded the responsibilities of child rearing and parenthood. This new experience of insomnia lasted quite some time and abated only with the intervention of psychotherapy as well as antidepressant medication.

Rachel's problems reveal an important ingredient in any true and, especially, chronic insomnia condition—that is, the condition of severe dependency is integrally tied to problems of sleep and of insomnia. Interestingly enough, people who are extremely dependent tend to sleep too much, especially when they are involved in relationships with caring partners who tend to gratify dependency cravings. In contrast, another way of understanding this idea is to equate intense dependency needs with immaturity and to consider that a person who has had such strong dependency needs frustrated will develop clinical symptoms of anxiety, depression, irritability, and insomnia.

> A young woman of 27 who was exceedingly dependent on her parents and husband would sleep far more than seemed to be necessary. She would retire in the early evening and, at times, not awaken until 1:00 or 2:00 P.M. the next day. This 15- or 16-hour slumber became the cause for much strife when her husband began complaining about her sleeping habits. As it turned out, her unusual hibernations were an effect both of a strongly developed dependency and of her resentment about it.
>
> Her prolonged sleeps were escape maneuvers from the real world—as she would say, from the "adult world." As her marriage began to dissolve, she became more and more vigilant at night until she began to experience bouts of insomnia. When her marriage finally ended, she was a full-fledged insomniac.

Thus, experiences in which dependency needs are gratified in relationships, as well as experiences of separation from these relationships, can profoundly affect the nature of one's sleep.

Persons who suffer with attachment and dependency problems may always entertain doubts about relationships. These doubts can be especially troublesome when a current relationship is about to dissolve. The overly dependent, overcontrolled person may want to go to sleep because, in the absence of support from others, deep inferiority feelings about doing things alone can cause intense anxiety. The dependent, undercontrolled person may not be able to sleep because the end of a relationship can be a dreadful reminder of always having been alone. In either case, dependency needs are overwhelming. They can lead to the experience of depressive feelings. The depression may become visible when a relationship fails—that is, at the point of separation when these dependency needs are frustrated. People who experience such problems, therefore, usually consider the formation or actual existence of a relationship to be the only corresponding means for the relief of depression and anxiety.

In the personality of the dependent, overattached person, as well as in the personality of the dependent underattached person, there reside the elements of eventual sleep problems because sleeping expresses the symbol of being *with* someone. It is the whole process of attachment that is intimately connected to relationships and to sleep. Even in sleep, individuals are object-related.

Narcolepsy and Dependency

The person with narcolepsy will be physiologically predisposed to it. Yet certain personality features can intensify this disorder and facilitate the appearance of narcoleptic symptoms. All of the narcoleptic patients described in this book reported early childhood experiences during which they were unnecessarily babied or else treated as though they were unimportant. This kind of childhood rearing practice unfortunately can be achieved in many different ways. Some of these patients were patronized while others were simply badgered with instructions and criticism. Such practices discouraged independent behavior and reinforced inordinate dependency needs. It is not uncommon for such persons to remember parents continually saying, "Never mind, you don't understand," "I'll take care of it," or any other such typical instruction indicating that the child is not well enough equipped to manage usual day-to-day problems.

Children who have based their understanding of attachment on these experiences can begin to feel profoundly inadequate and can grow up actually feeling unable to confront adult problems in adult ways. Such persons can also become guarded and may develop sarcastic and other angry ways to behave in order to guard against underlying vulnerability. They frequently believe that they cannot *do* things and they prefer to have someone else accomplish tasks for them. Thus, such people experience self-esteem problems and may consistently seek to reinforce intensely dependent needs.

This sort of dependency problem may be constructed in ways that make it seem impossible to solve. How can one hope to eliminate dependency needs that are based upon a lifelong conviction that one's basic survival is tied to another. Since such a dependent person, in addition, actually may not have been given any tacit permission to do things, or even to believe that they could be done, how can such a person not feel vulnerable and why should such a person not be guarded? In order not to be guarded or distrustful about relationships, a great deal of transformational therapeutic experience needs to be internalized so that enough ego-strength and the capacity to be assertive can be developed. This task is not an easy one because severe dependency produces many serious relationship problems. First, persons who have this problem may become inordinately demanding and defensive in order to conceal feelings of vulnerability. Such persons, therefore, can be highly resistive to therapy. Second, such persons may be quite inexperienced in social relationships, but need to appear mature; this, too, can interfere with relationships, including the therapy relationship. Finally, because of the presence of such strong needs for dependency as well as the presence of a sense of social awkwardness, such persons may deny and avoid all aggressive and competitive struggles. What may occur as a result of these problems is that repeated failures become a sort of behavioral signature of such people. Dependency is so great that little, if any, independent behavior occurs and failure experiences become typical. For the most part, such persons want all accomplishments to be achieved only in collaboration with and with the approval of the parent figure.

In the case of a therapy relationship, the therapist becomes the parent figure.

In a sense, a new *bringing up* needs to be aimed for—one in which this kind of person may freely express needs, dissatisfactions and feelings of all sorts and begin to *do* things in life. This *doing* must draw a sharp contrast between deeds and words. The doing must be seen as independent personal accomplishment. It must reflect solid achievement—the cornerstone of actual self-esteem internalization. In a psychotherapy setting, this new *bringing up* has a chance to develop. This point of a new bringing up is also discussed by Balint (1968).

Thus, for the narcoleptic, so-called reconstructive therapy work with respect to dependency needs means a rebuilding of certain aspects of personality structure so that the relationship with the world no longer resembles the early relationship with the "You can't do it—only I can do it" parent. Some of the issues that have to be dealt with in therapy include problems centering around attachment, dependency, assertiveness, social immaturity, and the need such persons may have for repeated failure experiences. Personality features of the narcoleptic patient corresponding to those described here have also been proposed in earlier papers by Barker (1948), Orthello, Langworthy and Betz (1944), Palmer (1941), and Sours (1963).

Insomnia and Dependency

In dependent persons with insomnia, it is proposed that early childhood experiences were also characterized by inadequate attachments and the appearance of corresponding subsequent intense dependency needs. However, such dependency needs developed from a different set of circumstances than those arising from the experience of narcoleptic persons described above. Persons with insomnia may have had early family experiences with parental figures who were perhaps overly self-absorbed and not terribly affectionate or reassuring. Such parents may have expected their children to perform without very much supervision. Yet, surprisingly enough, it is also quite likely that such parents were still somehow able to convey their love. These are not the kind of parents who either abused or hated their children.

Children of such parents are sometimes heard to say that they knew they were loved despite the absence of physical displays of affection.

> Diane, described in Chapter 10, always remembered her mother as a person who loved her, despite the fact that her mother was a very formal and perfectionistic woman. She would expect Diane to be able to do things well, but she hardly ever praised her.
>
> Diane grew up feeling a great need to depend on her mother. However, she also knew that her mother would never really meet this need.

Many persons with insomnia crave attachments that will guarantee caring and permanence in relationships. The assurance of permanence in some way replaces frustrated past needs for affection and love. Achieving decent relationships can help such persons become quite happy. When relationships terminate, however, insomnia—the condition of aloneness—can develop. To avoid this condition of aloneness, the person with insomnia will develop rigid coping styles in order not to feel completely isolated.

Children of formal and "objective" parents tend to develop rigid and guarded personality traits, as well as the tendency to be dissatisfied and distrustful. Such children may grow up feeling resistive to the world and resentful about an early lack of closer contact with parents. However, depending on how demanding early relationships actually were, such people may overtly behave in ways that appear to be quite competent and even socially agreeable. This agreeableness and pureness of intent are only apparent. Beneath the surface are highly guarded and ungiving personality inclinations reflecting a distrustful, rigid, and dissatisfied emotional disposition.

How can such people relinquish this distrustfulness? Better still, why should they? Without it, what can they expect? Historically, all such persons actually know about relationships is that they are characterized by the absence of total acceptance, they are demanding, and they expect precise performance. Persons with insomnia who have experienced this kind of early history dislike being considered distrustful and pessimistic, so they develop social skills and appearances of relatedness. They have been taught the lesson of alienation—never to depend on anyone emotionally. This sort of experience in life generates the idea that one may ask for things provided a good reason is supplied; one is, however, unjustified in asking for anything without reasons. It is a philosophy of life that teaches, "Hold on to whatever you have," because wanting something will not necessarily produce it. When such people actually find themselves in a satisfying and long-standing relationship, they usually have difficulty managing it despite the great importance they ascribe to it. Should such a relationship terminate, however, then severe insomnia may be expected to appear.

In summary, then, early dependency ties in persons with insomnia developed within the context of a relative absence of parental supervision, together with a continual hope for contact. In the therapy situation, the focus of sessions may be less on intellectual discussions and more on ventilating feelings of anger regarding an early sense of partial but significant deprivation. Therapy work for the insomniac concerns the development of a sense that to depend is permissible and can even be desirable, and that all relationships need not be depriving ones.

SEPARATION, INSOMNIA AND NARCOLEPSY

At any given time, the one major event that can evoke sensitive feelings about one's dependency needs is that of separation. For the narcoleptic person who is dependent, the possibility of separation usually means feeling extremely vulnerable. During times of separation, such a person may even appear detached as a way of concealing feelings of anxiety and depression. On the other hand, for the dependent person with insomnia, separation means that no longer can there be any hope of feeling close or of exchanging warm feelings with another person. The narcoleptic may use sleeping as an escape in order not to feel the separation. The insomniac perhaps cannot go to sleep because separation is so reminiscent of earlier experiences that it represents the expression of one's worst possible fears. Thus, for the insomniac, separation can be electrifying.

Separation for the dependent narcoleptic person means being in the dark. In the dark one sleeps. For the dependent person with insomnia, separation electrifies and this means to be in the light. In the light, one remains awake. For the narcoleptic person, the thought of losing a significant person means that the one who knows what to do and how to handle things is gone. Without such a person around to shed light on life, darkness falls. With nothing to do and with a sense of incapacity to match it, one sleeps.

For the insomniac, the thought of losing a significant person signifies that one's lifelong existential fear of loneliness has arrived. This congruence of fantasy and reality is so blatant that it can make the heart pound. "I knew it, I knew it, I knew it," might be the refrain, "no one is there." For both the narcoleptic person and the person with insomnia, separation experiences generate depression, anxiety, grief, and an overall defensive posture. However, the main emotions experienced by persons who have these sleep disorders are fear and anger.

Experiences of separation will always generate intense emotion which may or may not be experienced directly. For the narcoleptic, separation tends to produce a sense of fear or dread because of the sudden loss and the apprehension of "going it alone" and because the dependency need was so great in the first place that a sense of rage or even outrage may develop at the mere thought of being so abandoned.

Similarly for the insomniac, separation confirms one aspect of early dependency conditions—that of abandonment. Separation releases a mixture of anger and fear at the sudden recognition of earlier similar experiences. In these early experiences, the parental relationship was in some respects also characterized by emotional abandonment.

Most psychoanalysts would agree that both separation experiences and intense dependency needs breed fear and anger. What this means is that the fear of abandonment is usually more profoundly underscored by intense anger. A good example of the connection between separation and fear and anger can be observed in the behavior of chimpanzees that are sometimes kept as pets. When tame, dependent chimpanzees are even temporarily abandoned, they sometimes scream with fear as well as anger and will even fall to the ground trembling.

A paradoxical situation exists with dependent people who experience the sleep disorders of insomnia and narcolepsy. This paradox may be described as one in which separation events generate fear and anger; the anger reinforces further attachment needs; thereby making the separation all the more painful. What this means is that feelings of anger reinforce attachment needs because the anger is a response to having needs for contact frustrated; it is not anger of some primitive instinct of destruction. When someone is angry about being left alone, greater focus is thereby directed upon the need for attachment.

Thus, in dependent persons with insomnia and narcolepsy, attachment and dependency needs can be extremely intense. The frustration of these needs can breed rage which in turn increases the need for dependence. When no one is there to meet such needs, then genuine anguish and great tension and depression may occur. In many such people, the expression of these frustrations appears in the form of sleep problems—that is, either in narcoleptic-like going to sleep or insomnia.

CULTURAL DIFFERENCES WITH RESPECT TO SLEEP AND THE EVENTS OF SEPARATION AND LOSS

There are distinct cultural differences among peoples of the world in the treatment of loss, separation or death (Mead, 1950). Some cultures encourage immediate rituals characterized as a forgetting purge of the trauma. Others encourage active and prolonged mourning. It has been reported that in the Balinese culture people will go to sleep after the occurrence of some tragedy (Benedict, 1953). It may be that sleep is an offering of respect, but it also may symbolically reflect a communal show of solidarity with the departed person. For the Balinese, staying awake and mourning may symbolize the loss and separation. Sleeping can represent a defiance, a fraternal refusal to recognize the loss, or a show of solidarity.

Separation effects on people from all cultures are strong. No matter what rituals are invoked to ease the pain of separation, no matter how stoic one has been taught to be in times of crisis, if a significant relationship existed, then separation from it will have its devastating emotional effect (Hinton, 1967; Lindemann, 1944; Parkes, 1964; Peretz, 1970; Wretmark, 1959). This effect may be seen overtly, but if it is not, then it will surely cause internal emotional problems. It may be that those cultures that encourage a stoic management of separation will not be as adaptive or will not survive as well as those that encourage some emotional display. Apparently, it is beneficial to ventilate those feelings that are generated from problems of dependency and separation in order to ameliorate problems of sleep.

The treatment of individuals with narcolepsy or insomnia as described in this volume has been discussed with respect to several intervention modalities. These have included individual psychotherapy, group psychotherapy, short-term clinical consultation, in-hospital diagnostic and management service, as well as special ambulatory care, usually in the form of pharmacological treatment. In the final chapter of the book, the vicissitudes of these sleep disorders as they appear in specific family members and affect their relationships with one another shall be traced within the context of family therapy treatment. An unusual case of a sleep disordered family will be presented; most of the historical, familial, psychodynamic and overall theoretical issues that have been discussed throughout this volume will be revealed in the course of the treatment.

Chapter 16

A Sleep Disordered Family

A sleep disorder in a family member may become as much of an entrenched pathological family symptom as any other more conventional neurotic symptom. As a matter of fact, sleep disorders in individuals may ultimately prove to be especially responsive to family therapy intervention because of the specific psychological triggers inherent in individuals who experience such sleep problems. These triggers of *dependency* and *separation anxiety* have been explored throughout this volume. They are psychological effects that were born and nourished precisely within the family context. Any treatment of families in which such issues play a pivotal role will, in all probability, create many palpable opportunities both for cathartic and bona fide transformational therapeutic work to occur.

In closing this book, therefore, a striking case of a sleep disordered family will be presented. This family consisted of an only son with narcolepsy, his mother, who was a frantic and highly energized insomniac, and his father, who was silent most of the time, awkward, and socially inept. The family treatment undertaken can illustrate the dynamic interplay of forces among individual family members with different kinds of sleep problems, and how the family dynamics reinforced such symptom formations. In addition, the powerful effect of family therapy on specific sleep symptoms can be appreciated.

THE FAMILY MEMBERS

Sophie, the mother, was 50. She was irrepressibly manic and would do whatever someone else needed to do instead of waiting for that person to do it themselves. She could do it faster anyway. Her son Alan, 27 years old, became narcoleptic when he was inducted into the army at the age of 22. Her husband, Mike, who was the silent type, apparently had very little to contribute to any ongoing interaction in the home. He was a hardworking man who was first employed as a computer programmer and many years later became president of the company. He was a successful businessman.

All his life Alan felt that he wanted to do things, to go places, to participate in sports and other normal activities. He felt, however, unable to initiate any independent action without his mother's approval and help. Alan's father was not the type you could ask to do things with and his mother was always preoccupied with her own projects. She treated both Alan and her husband with marvelous condescension. Alan's most vivid early memory is of his father, in a moment of rare liberation, turning to his mother who was in the midst of one of her tirades and asking her to sign some kind of document. Alan remembers that she just kept right on with her "ranting," not even acknowledging her husband's request. His father then said, "All you want from me is the bed . . . bitch."

Alan reported that he was not disturbed by this encounter. His father's outburst somehow felt correct to him. In fact, he felt that his mother never really considered either of them to be terribly important. She paid them only a kind of procedural or perfunctory respect —never, however, forgetting to remind Alan that his father was a highly successful man and could get things done. She also suggested that Alan was not like him, but rather took after her father who was "lazy and would just lie around the house."

Alan felt these barbs acutely but pretended not to hear them. He could not talk to his father about them. Alan grew up not doing much of anything while feeling extremely dependent upon his mother.

Sophie had always been a "pill popper." She was a rather superficial person and was constantly concerned with what others thought and about her overall image in the world. Her insomnia was the kind in which she would awaken in the middle of the night when everyone else would be asleep. She also complained of many aches and pains but refused to do anything about them except ingest aspirin and sleep medication.

This family finally came for treatment only after Alan had, after several years of job hunting, become unemployable. He hated his father's business and refused to work in the factory. He was having sleep attacks and had had cataplectic attacks on his last job. The family sought treatment when their family physician suggested that it would be advisable for the entire family to seek family therapy.

Sophie

When the family started treatment, Sophie felt worse than ever. She viewed the treatment as an element in her life that was changing things and she became somewhat depressed and angry. She may even have perceived the treatment situation to be one that implied a sort of *separation* occurring in the typical patterns of the family interaction. At first Sophie was only moderately talkative and appeared soft-spoken and calm. After a while she became the family storyteller and would take over almost all conversation. At times Alan would try to stop her. More often, the therapist would have to redirect the discussion so that Alan or Mike could participate. Sophie would become annoyed at these interruptions and, as soon as she sensed that her role as the "family switchboard operator" was threatened, she created various difficulties about being able to attend the family therapy sessions. At one point, she almost succeeded in pulling the entire family out of treatment.

It was necessary for Sophie to continue to view Alan as the patient. After awhile she was no longer certain who the patient was. Was it Alan, was it Mike, or was it herself? The answer, which became increasingly clear, was that the patient was the entire family.

Sophie's insomnia and her anxious style of behavior were very much related to Mike's apparent detachment. For Sophie, Mike's silent ways reminded her of her father who always expected her to do things well, but who never really responded to her. Sophie was always canvassing Mike for affection and sexual contact. Her main anxiety was concerned with wondering whether Mike really loved her. She was usually angry about his silent presence because it made her feel that he was separate. When she would awaken each night, her difficulty in getting back to sleep revolved around thoughts of Mike's detachment. She would lie there each night with a full-blown attack of insomnia, feeling frightened, anxious and angry.

Sophie's relationship to Alan was problematic because she would compulsively remind him of his father's competence and success, but would conspicuously avoid discussing Mike's obvious detachment. She further showed her insensitivity towards Alan by telling him that he could not get things done and that she did everything for him.

Sophie described some of this material in the sessions in a tone that was accusing; she accused Alan of being inadequate, and Mike for his silence. Sophie's typical behavior in the sessions seemed defensive. It appeared as though she felt the family problems were her fault, and she used a good offensive-accusing posture to defend herself. Of course, the family interaction itself was problematic and this state of affairs was no one person's responsibility. However, Sophie quite readily assumed the implicit blame for all that was wrong in the family; in this, both Mike and Alan agreed.

Mike

Mike was a shy and socially isolated person and yet these qualities did not prevent him from succeeding in his professional life. Sophie said he married her because she was a lively person and thus complemented his lack of social grace. In addition, Mike eventually admitted that his love for Sophie was originally based on how she would unabashedly adore him.

Mike never admitted to having any sleep problems and resented both Sophie's insomnia and Alan's narcolepsy. He was, in fact, very disappointed with Alan; even though he tried to hide these feelings, his anger or irritation about Alan's apparent incapacities would frequently be obvious. Whenever Mike expressed any dissatisfaction with Alan, Sophie would intervene and try to protect Alan. However, whenever Alan tried to talk to his father or ask his advice about something, Mike would become visibly happy.

Mike was a self-made man and Sophie made sure that everyone knew it. In the sessions when Sophie would refer to Mike's success, he would always seem to appreciate her comments, especially because they gave him a sense of importance. Yet Mike would never favor Sophie with anything even resembling a verbal thank-you.

One of the highly neurotic components of this family's interaction was the reverence accorded Mike. He was on a very high pedestal and Sophie made sure he stayed up there. Alan was most affected by his father's position and he firmly believed that it would be impossible ever to match his father's success. Mike, on the other hand relished his elevated position and, in a peculiar way, it gave his silence in the family, a reason to exist.

Alan

An immature, well-meaning, yet hostile and overdependent boy is the way Alan might be described, despite the fact that he was 27 years old when the family came for therapy. He was somewhat depressed, was narcoleptic and was hopelessly unemployed. It seemed that he was constantly trying to control his mother's behavior. During the first phase of family meetings, he would always have at least one eye on her. He did this in order to gauge her mood and perhaps pick up some clues from her with respect to regulating his own behavior in the sessions.

Alan was virtually without friends. He spent his days sauntering through the house, sitting in his room, watching T.V., and sleeping on and off. He would have at least a half dozen narcoleptic sleep attacks each day. It was quite difficult for the family to talk about his narcolepsy, but Alan could talk about it endlessly. He was thoroughly interested in every aspect of it and was able to describe his narcoleptic symptoms in the greatest detail. He was quite bright and his dry wit was just a shade from being sarcastic or even cruel.

In the therpay sessions, he would infuriate his mother and seemed to enjoy opposing her. He would usually wait for her to make some inflated point about how much she was suffering and then would abruptly deflate her by mentioning some contradictory event. Even though Alan desperately needed her love and support, he nevertheless directed all of his anger toward her.

THE THERAPY SESSIONS

At first Sophie was watchful and timid. Alan was worried about this because he knew that his mother was not really the silent type and certainly not a calm person. Alan was apparently frightened that he would not be able to function without her overbearing and gratuitous supervision.

The family as a whole was rigid in its response to the presence of a therapist during the first few sessions. Alan would talk only to to his mother, Mike would simply try to be informational—that is, he would offer information to clarify points—while Sophie was only moderately involved although clearly the spokesperson for the family. Once the typical pattern of communication was established by the family, it was going to be the task and aim of the therapy to try and open it up so that newer and healthier patterns could be tried.

This family's problem—one that is not uncommon in most families—was that a particular style of communicating that existed between family members automatically eliminated the possibility of other styles developing. The communication of this family was a perfect example of such rigidity. Sophie ran the switchboard and both Alan and Mike conducted their communication through her. As the therapist continued to test the strength of this pattern, he instructed members to try to alter their patterns in specific ways. For example, Sophie would invariably start each session by raising an issue or by telling or recounting an event. Then Alan would say something and occasionally Mike would clarify it. Sophie would then agree with Mike —unless he criticized Alan—and her agreement sealed the end of the pattern, as it were. The pattern was always initiated by Sophie; Mike would eventually *help* Alan clarify something, and Sophie would agree with Mike's helpful comment. Alan, therefore, was always being helped. He could not ever say anything independently without some so-called helpful addition from Sophie or Mike.

Actually, Allan's anger was always directed towards Sophie because he felt both so controlled by her and so dependent on her. It soon became obvious that Alan's anger toward Sophie was really his father's proxy. What this meant was that Mike was the one who hardly ever directed any anger toward members of the family. Alan became Mike's voice in the family and this substitution process was one of the most neurotic patterns of the family. Sophie would talk to Mike through Alan, and Mike would express his sentiments toward Sophie also through Alan, but no one knew they were responding in this indirect manner.

When it was suggested that it would be important for someone other than Sophie to initiate each communication simply because it wasn't fair to place the entire burden of the therapy session on her, the family could not, at first, do it. Awkward silences followed and before anyone knew it, somehow Sophie was saying something and Alan was replying, or Sophie would start by saying, "Well, someone else has to start, right?" It was apparently very difficult for the family to alter its basic interactional style.

THE CENTRAL PROBLEM

The most neurotic element in the family concerned the nature of each person's mixed or ambivalent feelings toward the other members. Each member of the family was intensely dependent on another member and was simultaneously very angry toward the one they were dependent upon. Sophie adored Mike but she felt deprived because he ignored her. Her insomnia was filled with rage towards him. Mike needed Sopie's sociability to add color to his life, but he also hated her controlling behavior. Alan was practically unable to function without Sophie but he never missed an opportunity to throw barbs at her or to expose her weaknesses. Mike was quite critical towards Alan, as was Sophie, except that Sophie would protect Alan from Mike's criticism. Nevertheless, Mike needed Alan, especially because Alan frequently irritated Sophie, and Sophie also needed Alan to compensate for the lack of contact she had with Mike. Everyone needed everyone else and everyone was correspondingly angry with everyone else. The dependency needs were so intense in this family that they generated anger in all directions. The anger, in turn, simply reinforced the dependency as well as the typical neurotic interactional family style. This sort of neurotic circuit had to be changed if the various family members were to be helped. The main problem was to help members reduce their dependency cravings without raising separation fears.

CHANGING

Gradually, Mike began to ask more questions. This became especially noticeable when Alan described his drowsiness at length. Apparently, Alan had never before discussed his narcolepsy with his father. Mike then described how, during his own adolescence, he too, used to be drowsy both during and after school. He also said that even up to the present time he likes to take naps in the middle of the day and does so in his office. Furthermore, he remembered that his own mother had, in hushed tones, told about one of her parents who used to fall in the streets with what was thought to be epilepsy.

Mike would not say very much more about this but Alan was stunned. He instantly knew that this great-grandparent was having cataplectic attacks and not epileptic ones. All of them were flabbergasted by this bit of information. It was not clear whether Mike had always seen the connection between Alan's narcolepsy and his grandparent's problem or whether he had suppressed the connection and would be angry at Alan as a way of distancing himself from ever seeing it. In any event, no one asked Mike why he had never before revealed this stunning bit of information.

After this revelation, Alan and his father began to talk more to each other. Alan also became noticeably less hostile toward his mother and, in an overall way, less sarcastic. Mike's hidden drowsiness and obvious silences began to appear to be similar to narcoleptic personality features of withdrawal and isolation. As a matter of speculation, Mike may have had minor narcoleptic personality effects without actually ever having developed any classic narcoleptic symptoms.

The sessions produced significant changes in each of the participants. Over a six-month period they began to gradually talk to each other instead of each addressing the therapist separately. Alan complained to his mother that she babied him and actually told his father that he wished he would talk more. Mike, indeed, began talking both to Alan and Sophie. Sophie—well, Sophie was interesting. She complained that Alan's dependency was draining her energies and that Mike's silence scared her to death. Everyone seemed to be truly enlightened and even friendlier as a result of these newly spoken revelations. Sophie's insomnia significantly subsided and Alan's sleep attacks also decreased.

At the beginning of therapy, all of the attitudes and emotions experienced by persons with insomnia and narcolepsy seemed to be dancing around the room. These included paranoid distrustfulness and hysterical susceptibility, depression, anger and fear, attachment needs and separation anxieties, severe dependency needs, and insomnia and narcolepsy proper. After some time, however, instead of feeling neurotically dependent and terrified of separation, this family began to feel they were healthier and together—a beginning.

Thus, although sleep disorders such as narcolepsy and insomnia are experienced by individuals, they may also be treated within a family framework. The important point to remember, however, is that sleep disorders—especially in dependent personalities—will be integrally tied to the broad issue of the nature of relationships and to the specific experience of separation. Sleep disorders, therefore, may be accurately called phenomena of separation.

References

AGNEW, H. W. JR. and WEBB, W. B. The sleep patterns of long and short sleepers. Paper presented at the meeting of the Association for the Psychophysiological Study of Sleep, Santa Monica, Cal., 1967.

AGNEW, H., WEBB, W. and WILLIAMS, R. The effect of stage 4 sleep deprivation. *Electroencephalography and Clinical Neurophysiology*, 1964, 17, 68.

AKERT, K. The anatomical substrate of sleep. *Progress in Brain Research,* 1965, 18: 9.

ANDERS, T. F. and GUILLEMINAULT, C. The pathophysiology of sleep disorders in pediatrics. In: Schulman, I. (Ed.), *Advances in pediatrics.* Vol. 22. Year Book Medical Publishers, Chicago, 1976.

ASERINSKY, E. and KLEITMAN, N. Regularly occurring periods of eye motility and concomitant phenomena during sleep. *Science,* 1953, 118: 273-274.

BAEKELAND, F. and HARTMANN, E. Sleep requirements and the characteristics of some sleepers. In: Hartmann, E. (Ed.), *Sleep and dreaming.* Boston: Little Brown and Company, 1970.

BALDY-MOULINIER, M., ARGUNER, A., and BESSET, A. Ultradian and circadian rhythms in sleep and wakefulness. In: Guilleminault, C., Dement, W. C., and Passouant, P. (Eds.), *Narcolepsy: Advances in sleep research, Vol. 3.* New York: Spectrum Publications, 1976.

BALINT, M. *The basic fault.* London: Tavistock Publications, 1968 (Reissued: New York: Brunner/Mazel, 1979).

Ban, T. A. *Psychopharmacology.* Baltimore: Williams and Wilkins, 1969.

BARKER, W. Studies in epilepsy: personality pattern, situational stress and symptoms in narcolepsy. *Psychosomatic Medicine,* 1948, 10:193-202.

BENEDICT, R. *Patterns of culture.* New York: The New American Library, 1953.

BERGER, R. J. and OSWALD, I. Effects of sleep deprivation on behavior, subsequent sleep and dreaming. *Journal of Mental Science,* 1962, 108: 454-465.

BERGMAN, A. "I" and "you": the separation-individuation process in the treatment of a symbiotic-psychotic child. In: McDevitt, J. B. and Settlage, C. F. (Eds.), *Separation-individuation.* New York: International Universities Press, 1971.

BEUTLER, L. E., THORNBY, J. I., and KARACAN, I. Psychological variables in the diagnosis of insomnia. In: Williams, R. L. and Karacan, I. (Eds.), *Sleep disorders: Diagnosis and treatment.* New York: John Wiley, 1978.

BIXLER, E. O., KALES, J. D., SCHARF, M. B., et al. Incidence of sleep disorders in medical practice; a physician survey. *Sleep Research,* 1976, 5: 160.

BLISS, E. Sleep in schizophrenia and depression: studies of sleep loss in man and animals. *Res. Publ. Ass. Nerv. Ment. Dis.,* 1967, 45: 195.

BONDUELLE, M. and DEGOS, C. Symptomatic narcolepsies: a critical study. In: Guilleminault, C., Dement, W. C., and Passouant, P. (Eds.), *Narcolepsy: Advances in sleep research, Vol. 3.* New York: Spectrum Publications, 1976.

BONSTEDT, T. Emotional aspects of the narcolepsies. *Disorders of the Nervous System.* October, 1954, 10, 291-299.

BOWLBY, J. *Attachment and loss: Separation,* Vol. II. New York: Basic Books, 1973.

BROCK, S. and WIESEL, B. The narcoleptic-cataplectic syndrome—an excessive and dissociated reaction of the sleep mechanism—and its accompanying mental states. *Journal of Nervous and Mental Disease,* 1941, 94: 700-712.

BROUGHTON, R. and GHANEM, P. The impact of compound narcolepsy on the life of the patient. In: Guilleminault, C., Dement, W. C., and Passouant, P. (Eds.), *Narcolepsy: Advances in sleep research, Vol. 3.* New York: Spectrum Publications, 1976.

BROUGHTON, R. and MAMELAK, M. Gamma-Hydroxy-Butyrate in the treatment of narcolepsy: a preliminary report. In: Guilleminault, C., Dement, W. C., and Passouant, P. (Eds.), *Narcolepsy: Advances in sleep research, Vol. 3.* New York: Spectrum Publications, 1976.

CADILHAC, J. Tricyclics and REM sleep. In: Guilleminault, C., Dement, W. C., and Passouant, P. (Eds.), *Narcolepsy: Advances in sleep research, Vol. 3.* New York: Spectrum Publications, 1976.

COHN, R. and CRUVANT, B. A. Relation of narcolepsy to the epilepsies. *Archives of Neurological Psychiatry,* 1944, 51: 163-170.

CONROY, R. and MILLS, J. N. *Human circadian rhythms.* Baltimore: Williams and Wilkins, 1971.

COODLEY, A. Psychodynamic factors in narcolepsy and cataplexy. *Psychiatric Quarterly,* 1948, 22: 596.

COOPER, J. R. (Ed.), Sedative-hypnotic drugs: risks and benefits. Rockville, Md.: National Institute on Drug Abuse, United States Department of Health, Education and Welfare, 1977.

DALY, D. and YOSS, R. A family with narcolepsy. *Proceedings of Staff Meetings, Mayo Clinic,* 1959, 34: 313-320.

DAVISON, C. Psychological and psychodynamic aspects of disturbances in sleep mechanisms. *Psychoanalytic Quarterly,* 1945, 14: 478.

DEMENT, W. C. The effect of dream deprivation. *Science,* 1960, 131: 1705-1707.

DEMENT, W. C. Recent studies on the biological role of rapid eye movement sleep. *American Journal of Psychiatry,* 1965, 122: 404-408.

DEMENT, W. C. *Some must watch while some must sleep.* San Francisco: W. H. Freeman Co., 1972.

DEMENT, W. CARSKADON, M. and LEY, R. The prevalence of narcolepsy, II. In: Chase, M. H., Stern, W. C., and Walter, P. L. (Eds.), *Sleep research,* Vol. 2. Los Angeles: Brain Information Service/Brain Research Institute, UCLA, 1973.

DEMENT, W. C. and KLEITMAN, N. The relation of eye movements during sleep to dream activity; an objective method for the study of dreaming. *Journal of Experimental Psychology,* 1957, 53: 339-346.

DEMENT, W. C. and MITLER, M. M. New developments in the basic mechanisms of sleep. In: Usdin, G. (Ed.), *Sleep research and clinical practice*. New York: Brunner/Mazel, 1973.

DEMENT, W., RECHTSCHAFFEN, A. and GULEVICH, G. The nature of the narcoleptic sleep attack. *Neurology*, 1966, 16: 18-33.

DERMAN, S. and KARACAN, I. Sleep-induced respiratory disorders. *Psychiatric Annals*, 1979, 9: 41-61.

Diagnostic classification of sleep and arousal disorders. Association of Sleep Disorder Centers, First edition, prepared by the Sleep Disorders Classification Committee, H. P. Roffwarg, Chairman, *Sleep*, 2:1-137, 1979.

DRAKE, F. Narcolepsy: Brief review and report of cases. *American Journal of Medical Science*, 1949, 218: 101-114.

EILENBERG, D. and WOODS, L. Narcolepsy with psychosis: report of two cases. *Proceedings of Staff Meetings, Mayo Clinic*, 1962, 37:561-566.

EPHRON, H. S. and CARRINGTON, P. Rapid eye movement sleep and cortical homeostasis. *Psychological Review*, 1966, Vol. 73, No. 6, 500-526.

ERIKSON, E. *Childhood and society*. Second Edition, New York: Norton, 1963.

ETHELBERG, S. Symptomatic "cataplexy" or chalastic fits in cortical lesion of the frontal lobe. *Brain*, 1950, 73: 499-512.

ETHELBERG, S. Sleep-paralysis or postdormitial chalastic fits in cortical lesions of the frontal pole. *Acta Psychiatrica et Neurologica Scandinavica Suppl*. 1956, 108: 121-130.

EVERETT, H. C. Sleep paralysis in medical students. *Journal of Nervous and Mental Disease*, 1963, 136: 283-287.

FARBER, I. J. Clinical symposium psychotherapy of a patient with narcolepsy. *Journal of the Hillside Hospital*, Jan. 1962, XII, 1:29-56.

FEINBERG, I. and HIATT, J. H. Sleep patterns in schizophrenia: a selective review. In: Williams, R. L. and Karacan, I. (Eds.), *Sleep disorders: Diagnosis and treatment*. New York: John Wiley, 1978.

FISCHGOLD, H., LAVERNHE, J. and BLANC, C. Sleep, insomnia and sleep debt in aeronautical medicine. *Presse Medicale*, February 1967.

FODOR, N. *The search for the beloved*. New York: Hermitage Press Inc., 1949.

FREUD, S. Dostoevsky and parricide. In: Strachey, J. (Ed.), *The complete psychological works of Sigmund Freud*. Standard Edition, 21, 1961, London: Hogarth Press, Originally published 1927.

FREUD, S. The ego and the id. In: Strachey, J. (Ed.), *The complete psychological works of Sigmund Freud*. Standard Edition, 19, 1961, London: Hogarth Press, Originally published 1923.

FREUD, S. The interpretation of dreams. In: Strachey, J. (Ed.), *The complete psychological works of Sigmund Freud. Standard Edition*, 4, 5, 1953, London: Hogarth Press, Originally published 1900.

GANADO, W. The narcolepsy syndrome. *Neurology*, 1958, 8: 487.

GÉLINEAU, J. B. De la narcolepsie. *Gaz. d'Hop*. 1880, 54: 635-637.

GILL, M. M. and BRENMAN, M. *Hypnosis and related states*. New York: International Universities Press, Inc., 1959.

GLOBUS, G. G. Sleep duration and feeling state. In: Hartmann, E. (Ed.), *Sleep and dreaming*. Boston: Little Brown and Company, 1970.

GOODE, G. B. Sleep paralysis. *Archives of Neurology*, 1962, 6: 228-234.

GREENBERG, R. Dream interruption insomnia. *Journal of Nervous and Mental Disease*, 967, 144: 1, 18-21.

GUILLEMINAULT, C. Cataplexy. In: Guilleminault, C., Dement, W. C., and Passonant,

P. (Eds.), *Narcolepsy: Advances in sleep research, Vol. 3.* New York: Spectrum Publications, 1976.

GUILLEMINAULT, C. Narcolepsy. In: Guilleminault, C., Dement, W. C., and Passonant P. (Eds.), *Narcolepsy Advances in sleep research, Vol. 3.* New York: Spectrum Publications, 1976.

GUILLEMINAULT, C. and DEMENT, W. C. Sleep apnea syndromes and related sleep disorders. In: Williams, R. L. and Karacan, I. (Eds.), *Sleep disorders: Diagnosis and treatment.* New York: John Wiley, 1978.

GUILLEMINAULT, C., ELDRIDGE, F. L., and DEMENT, W. C. Insomnia with sleep apnea: a new syndrome. *Science,* 1973, 181: 856-858.

GULEVICH, G., DEMENT, W., and JOHNSON, I. Psychiatric and EEG observations on a case of prolonged (26 hours) wakefulness. *Archives of General Psychiatry,* 1966, 15: 29-35.

GUNTRIP, H. *Schizoid phenomena, object relations, and the self.* New York: International Universities Press, 1968.

GUPTA, B. and DEKA, D. Application of chronobiology to radiotherapy of tumor of oral cavity. *Chronobiologia,* 1975, 2: 25.

GUTHEIL, E. *The handbook of dream analysis.* New York: Liveright Publishing Corp., 1951.

HALBERG, F. et al. Autorhythmometry procedures for physiologic self-measurement and their analysis. *Physiology Teacher,* 1972, 1: 1-11.

HARLOW, H. The nature of love. Presidential address delivered at the American Psychological Association, Washington, D.C., August, 1958, and printed in the *American Psychologist,* 1958, 13: 673-685.

HARTMANN, E. *The biology of dreaming.* Springfield, Illinois: C. C Thomas, 1967.

HARTMANN, E. What is good sleep? In: Hartmann, E. (Ed.), *Sleep and dreaming,* Boston: Little Brown & Co., 1970.

HARTMANN, E. Long term administration of psychotropic drugs: effects on human sleep. In: Williams, R. L. and Karacan, I. (Eds.), *Pharmacology of sleep.* New York: John Wiley, 1976.

HAURI, P. What is good sleep? In: Hartmann, E. (Ed.), *Sleep and dreaming.* Boston: Little Brown & Co., 1970.

HAURI, P., and HAWKINS, D. R. Alpha-delta sleep. *Electroencephalography and Clinical Neurophysiology,* 1973, 34: 233-237.

HAWKINS, D. R. Implications of knowledge of sleep patterns in psychiatric conditions. In: Hartmann, E. (Ed.), *Sleep and dreaming,* Boston: Little Brown & Co., 1970.

HAWKINS, D. R. Depression and sleep research: basic science and clinical perspective. In: Usdin, G. (Ed.), *Depression: Clinical, biological, and psychological perspectives.* New York: Brunner/Mazel, 1976.

HAWKINS, D. R. Sleep and depression. *Psychiatric Annals,* August, 1979, 9, 8: 13-28.

HAWKINS, D. R. and MENDELS, J. Sleep disturbance in depressive syndromes. *American Journal of Psychiatry,* 1966, 123: 682.

HAWKINS, D. R. et al. The psychophysiology of sleep in psychotic depression: a longitudinal study. *Psychosomatic Medicine,* 1967, 29: 329-344.

HINTON, J. M. Patterns of insomnia in depressive states. *Journal of Neurosurgical Psychiatry,* 1963, 26: 184.

HINTON, J. *Dying.* Baltimore: Penguin Books, 1967.

HISHIKAWA, Y. Sleep paralysis. In: Guilleminault, C., Dement, W. C., and Passonant, P. (Eds.), *Narcolepsy: Advances in sleep research, Vol. 3.* New York: Spectrum Publications, 1976.

HISHIKAWA, Y., EIDA, H., NAKAR, K., and KANEKO, Z. Treatment of narcolepsy with imipramine (Tofranil) and desmethylimipramine (Pertofan). *Journal of Neurological Science,* 1966, 3: 453.

HOBSON, J. A. The cellular basis of sleep cycle control. *Advances in Sleep Research,* 1974, 1: 217-250.

HOLLIDAY, A. R. Review of psychopharmacology. In: Wolman, B. B. (Ed.), *Handbook of clinical psychology*. New York: McGraw Hill, 1965.

HONIGFELD, G., and HOWARD, A. *Psychiatric drugs.* New York: Academic Press, 1973.

JACOBSON, E. *The self and the object world.* New York: International Universities Press, 1964.

JELLIFFE, S. E. Narcolepsy; Hypnolepsy; Pkynolepsy. *Med. J. Rec.,* 1929, 129: 269. Cited in Wagner, C. P. Comment on the mechanism of narcolepsy; with case reports. *Journal of Nervous and Mental Disease,* 1930, 72: 405-416.

JONES, E. *On the nightmare*. London: Hogarth Press Ltd., 1949.

JONES, H. S. and OSWALD, I. Two cases of healthy insomnia. *Electroencephalography and Clinical Neurophysiology,* 1968, 35: 378-380.

KAHN, E. Age-related changes in sleep characteristics. In: Hartmann, E. (Ed.), *Sleep and dreaming*. Boston: Little Brown & Co., 1970.

KALES, A. (Ed.), *Sleep: Physiology and pathology*. Philadelphia: J. P. Lippincott Co., 1969.

KALES, A., BIXLER, E. O., TAN, T. L. et al. Chronic hypnotic drug use: ineffectiveness, drug withdrawal insomnia, and hypnotic drug dependence. *Journal of the American Medical Association,* 1974, 277: 513-517.

KALES, A., CALDWELL, A. B., PRESTON, T. A., et al. Personality patterns in insomnia. *Archives of General Psychiatry,* 1976, 33: 1128-1134.

KALES, A. and KALES, J. Sleep laboratory evaluation of psychoactive drugs. *Pharmacological Physicians,* 1970, 4: 1-6.

KALES, A. and KALES, J. Recent advances in the diagnosis and treatment of sleep disorders. In: Usdin, G. (Ed.), *Sleep research and clinical practice.* New York: Brunner/Mazel, 1973.

KALES, A., KALES, J. D. Sleep disorders: recent findings in the diagnosis and treatment of disturbed sleep. *New England Journal of Medicine,* 1974, 290: 487-499.

KALES, J. D., KALES, A., BIXLER, E. O., and SOLDATOS, C. R. Resource for managing sleep disorders. *Journal of the American Medical Association,* 1979, 241, 22: 2413-2416.

KALES, A. et al. Sleep patterns of a Pentobarbital addict before and after withdrawal. *Psychophysiology,* 1968, 5: 208.

KALES, A. et al. Sleep disturbances following sedative use and withdrawal. In: Kales, A. (Ed.), *Sleep: Physiology and pathology*. Philadelphia: J. P. Lippincott Co., 1969.

KALES, A. et al. Sleep patterns following 205 hours of sleep deprivation. *Psychosomatic Medicine,* 1970, 32: 189-200.

KALES, A. et al. Sleep patterns of insomniac subjects: further studies. *Psychophysiology,* 1972, 9: 137.

KALES, A. et al. Incidence of insomnia in the Los Angeles metropolitan area. Paper presented at the 14th Annual Meeting of the Association for the Psychophysiological Study of Sleep. Jackson Hole, Wyoming, 1974.

KALES, A. et al. Comparative effectiveness of nine hypnotic drugs: sleep laboratory studies. *Journal of Clinical Pharmacology,* 1977, 17: 207-213.

KARACAN, I., MOORE, C. A. and WILLIAMS, R. L. The narcoleptic syndrome. *Psychiatric Annals,* 1979, 9, 7: 69-76.

KARACAN, I. and WILLIAMS, R. L. Insomnia; Old wine in a new bottle. *Psychiatric Quarterly*, 1971, 45: 1-15.

KARACAN, I. et al. Prevalence of sleep disturbance in a primarily urban Florida county. *Social Scientific Medicine*, 1976, 10: 239-244.

KAY, D. C. et al. Human pharmacology of sleep. In: Williams, R. L. and Karacan, I. (Eds.), *Pharmacology of sleep*. New York: John Wiley & Sons, 1976.

KELLERMAN, H. Relating emotions and traits in the measurement of maladjustment. *Proceedings of the 73rd Annual Convention of the American Psychological Association*, 1965, 229-230.

KELLERMAN, H. The relation of suicidal acts to flight into health states. *Transnational Mental Health Research Newsletter*. 1976, XVIII, 2: 15-16.

KELLERMAN, H. *Group psychotherapy and personality: Intersecting structures*. New York: Grune & Stratton, 1979.

KELLERMAN, H. A structural model of emotion and personality: psychoanalytic and sociobiological implications. In: Plutchik, R. and Kellerman, H. (Eds.), *Emotion: Theory research and experience, Vol. 1, Theories of emotion*. New York: Academic Press, 1980.

KELLERMAN, H. and PLUTCHIK, R. Emotion-trait interrelations and the measurement of personality. *Psychological Reports*, 1968, 23: 1107-1114.

KERNBERG, O. F. Boundaries and structure in love relations. *Journal of the American Psychoanalytic Association*, 1977, 25: 81-114.

KESSLER, S. Genetic factors in narcolepsy. In: Guilleminault, C., Dement, W. C. and Passonant, P. (Eds.), *Narcolepsy: Advances in sleep research, Vol. 3*. New York: Spectrum Publications, 1976.

KING, C. D. The pharmacology of rapid eye movement sleep. *Advances in Pharmacology and Chemotherapy*, 1971, 9: 1-91.

KLEITMAN, N. *Sleep and wakefulness*, Chicago: University of Chicago Press, 1939, 1963.

KLEITMAN, N. Implications of the rest-activity cycle: implications for organization of activities. In: Hartmann, E. (Ed.), *Sleep and dreaming*. Boston: Little Brown and Co., 1970.

KLERMAN, G. L. and PAYKEL, E. S. The tricyclic antidepressants. In: Clark, W. G. and Giudice, J. del (Eds.), *Principles of psychopharmacology*. New York: Academic Press, 1970.

KOHUT, H. *The reconstruction of the self*. New York: International Universities Press, 1977.

KRABBE, E., and MAGNUSSEN, G. Familial narcolepsy. *Acta Psychiatrica Neurologica*, 1942, 17: 149-173.

KUPFER, D. J. A psychobiologic marker for primary depressive disease. *Biological Psychiatry*, 1976, 11: 159-174.

KUPFER, D. J. and FOSTER, F. G. The sleep of psychotic patients: Does it all look alike? In: Freedman, D. X. (Ed.), *Biology of the major psychoses: A comparative analysis*. Raven Press, 1975.

KUPFER, D. J. et al. Sleep disturbance in acute schizophrenic patients. *American Journal of Psychiatry*, 1970, 126: 47-57.

KUPFER, D. J. et al. The application of EEG sleep for the differential diagnosis of affective disorders. *American Journal of Psychiatry*, 1978, 135: 69-74.

KUPFERMANN, K. The development and treatment of a psychotic child. In: McDevitt, J. B. and Settlage, C. F. (Eds.), *Separation-individuation*. New York: International Universities Press, 1971.

LECKMAN, J. F. and GERSHON, E. S. A genetic model of narcolepsy. *British Journal of Psychiatry*, 1976, 128: 276-279.

LEVIN, M. Aggression, guilt, and cataplexy. *American Journal of Psychiatry*, 1953, 116: 133-136.

LIDDON, S. Sleep paralysis and hypnagogic hallucinations: their relationship to the nightmare. *Archives of General Psychiatry*, 1967, 17: 88-96.

LINDEMANN, E. Symptomatology and management of acute grief. *American Journal of Psychiatry*, 1944, 101: 141.

LUCE, G. G. *Body time*. New York: Random House, 1971.

LUCE, G. G. and SEGAL, J. *Insomnia*. New York: Doubleday & Co., 1969.

LUGARESI, E. Brief clinical and physiopathogenetic remarks on narco-cataplexic syndromes. *Electroencephalography and Clinical Neurophysiology*, 1961, 13: 136.

LUGARESI, E., COCCAGNA, G., MANTOVANI, M., and CIRIGNOTTA, F. Hypersomnia with periodic apnea. In: Guilleminault, C., Dement, W. C., and Passouant, P. (Eds.), *Narcolepsy: Advances in sleep research, Vol. 3*. New York: Spectrum Publications, 1976.

MAGOUN, H. An ascending reticular activating system in the brain stem. *Archives of Neurology and Psychiatry*, 1952, 67: 145-154.

MAGOUN, H. *The waking brain*. Springfield, Ill.: Charles C. Thomas, 1958.

MAHLER, M. S. *On human symbiosis and the viscissitudes of individuation*. New York: International Universities Press, 1968.

MAHLER, M., PINE, F., and BERGMAN, A. *The psychological birth of the human infant: Symbiosis and individuation*. New York: Basic Books, 1975.

MALITZ, S. Drug therapy: antidepressants. In: Arieti, S. (Ed.), *American handbook of psychiatry: Vol. 3*. New York: Basic Books, 1966.

MCKELLAR, P. and SIMPSON, L. Between wakefulness and sleep: hypnagogoic imagery. *British Journal of Psychology*, 1954, 45: 266-276.

MEAD, M. *Sex and temperament in three primitive societies*. New York: The New American Library, 1950.

MENDELS, J. and HAWKINS, D. R. Sleep and depression: a controlled EEG study. *Archives of General Psychiatry*, 1967, 16: 344-354.

MENDELS, J. and HAWKINS, D. R. Sleep and depression. IV Longitudinal studies. *Journal of Nervous and Mental Disease*, 1971, 153: 251-272.

MENDELSON, W. B., GILLIN, J. C. and WYATT, R. J. *Human sleep and its disorders*. New York: Plenum Press, 1977.

MILLS, J. N. Human circadian rhythms. *Physiological Review*, 1966, 40:128-165.

MISSRIEGLER, A. On the psychogenesis of narcolepsy: report of a case cured by psychoanalysis (tr. B. Karpman). *Journal of Nervous and Mental Disease*, 1941, 93: 141.

MITCHELL, S. A. and DEMENT, W. C. Narcolepsy syndrome: antecedent, contiguous, and concomitant nocturnal sleep disordering and deprivation. *Psychophysiology*, 1968, 4: 398.

MITCHELL, S. A., DEMENT, W. C. and GULEVICH, G. D. The so-called "ideopathic" narcolepsy syndrome. Paper presented at the Annual Meeting of the Association for the Psychophysiological Study of Sleep, Gainesville, Florida, March, 1966.

MITLER, M. Toward an animal model of narcolepsy-cataplexy. In: Weitzman, E. (Ed.), *Advances in sleep research*. New York: Spectrum Publications, 1976.

MOLLER, E. and OSTENFELD, I. Studies on the cerebral carotid syndrome and the physiological basis of consciousness. *Acta Psychiatrica Neurologica*, 1949, 24: 59-80.

MONROE, L. J. Psychological and physiological differences between good and poor sleepers. *Journal of Abnormal Psychology*, 1967, 72: 255-264.

MONTPLAISIR, J. Disturbed nocturnal sleep. In: Guilleminault, C., Dement, W. C., and Passouant, P. (Eds.), *Narcolepsy: Advances in sleep research, Vol. 3*. New York: Spectrum Publications, 1976.

MORGENSTERN, A. L. The neurotic component in narcolepsy. *American Journal of Psychiatry*, Sept. 1965, 122: 3, 306-312.

MORUZZI, G. and MAGOUN, H. W. Brain stem reticular formation and activation of the EEG. *Electroencephalography and Clinical Neurophysiology*, 1949, 1: 455-473.

NETTER, F. H. *The CIBA collection of medical illustrations: Vol. 1. The nervous system*. New York: Colorpress, 1968.

ORTHELLO, R., LANGWORTHY, R. and BETZ, B. J. Narcolepsy as a type of response to emotional conflicts. *Psychosomatic Medicine*, 1944, 6: 211-226.

OSWALD, I. Drugs and sleep *Pharmacological Review*, 1968, 20: 273-303.

OSWALD, I. Sleep dependence on amphetamine and other drugs. In: Kales, A. (Ed.), *Sleep: Physiology and pathology*. Philadelphia: J. B. Lippincott, 1969.

OSWALD, I. and PRIEST, R. G. Five weeks to escape the sleeping pill habit. *British Medical Journal*, 1965, 2: 1093-1099.

OSWALD, I. et al. Melancholia and barbiturates: a controlled EEG, body and eye movement study of sleep. *British Journal of Psychiatry*, 1963, 109: 66.

PALMER, H. Narcolepsy. *British Medical Journal*, 1941, 378.

PARENS, H. and SAUL, L. J. *Dependence in man*. New York: International Universities Press, 1971.

PARKES, C. M. Recent bereavement as a cause of mental illness. *British Journal of Psychiatry*, 1964, 110: 198.

PARKES, J. D. Amphetamines and alertness. In: Guilleminault, C., Dement, W. C., and Passouant, P. (Eds.), *Narcolepsy: Advances in sleep research, Vol. 3*. New York: Spectrum Publications, 1976.

PERETZ, D. Reaction to loss. In: Schoenberg, B., Carr, A. C., Peretz, D. and Kutscher, A. H. *Loss and grief*. New York: Columbia University Press, 1970.

PFLUG, B. and TOLLE, R. Disturbance of the 24-hour rhythm in endogenous depression and the treatment of endogenous depression by sleep deprivation. *International Journal of Pharmacopsychiatry*, 1971, 6: 187-196. (a)

PFLUG, B. and TOLLE, R. Therapy of endogenous depression by sleep deprivation: practical and theoretical consequences. *Nervenarzt*, 1971, 42: 117-124. (b)

Physicians desk reference. New York: Medical Economics, 1978.

PLUTCHIK, R. and KELLERMAN, H. *The emotions profile index: Test and manual*. Los Angeles: Western Psychological Services, 1974.

POND, D. A. Narcolepsy: a brief critical review and study of 8 cases. *Journal of Mental Science*, 1952, 98: 595-605.

PRUDOM, A. and KLEMM, W. Electrographic correlates of sleep behavior in a primitive mammal, the armadillo Dasypus noremcintus. *Physiological Behavior*, 1973, 10: 275-282.

RECH, R. H. and MOORE, K. F. (Eds.), *An introduction to psychopharmacology*. New York: Raven Press, 1971.

RECHTSCHAFFEN, A. and DEMENT, W. Studies on the relation of narcolepsy, cataplexy and sleep with low voltage random EEG activity. In: Ketz, S., Evarts, E. V. and Williams, H. W. (Eds.), *Sleep and altered states of consciousness*. Baltimore: Williams and Williams, 1967.

RECHTSCHAFFEN, A., WOLBERT, E., DEMENT, W. C., et al. Nocturnal sleep of narcoleptics. *Electroencephalography and Clinical Neurophysiology,* 1963, 15: 599-609.

RICHTER, C. P. *Biological clocks in medicine and psychiatry,* Springfield, Ill.: C. C. Thomas, 1965.

ROBERTS, H. J. Unrecognized narcolepsy and amphetamine abuse. *Medical Counterpoint,* August, 1979, 28-42.

ROTH, B. Narcolepsy and hypersomnia. In: Williams, R. L. and Karacan, I. (Eds.), *Sleep disorders: Diagnosis and treatment.* New York: John Wiley & Sons, 1978.

ROTH, B., BRUHOVA, S. and LEHOVSKY, M. On the problem of pathophysiological mechanisms of narcolepsy, hypersomnia and dissociated sleep disturbances. In: Gastaut, H., Lugaresi, E., Berti, C., Ceroui, G., and Coccagna, G. (Eds.), *The abnormalities of sleep in man.* Bologna: Aulo Gaggi, 1968.

SAMPSON, H. Psychological effects of deprivation of dreaming sleep. *Journal of Nervous and Mental Disease,* 1966, 143: 305-317.

SARBIN, T. R. and COE, W. C. *Hypnosis.* New York: Holt, Rinehart and Winston, Inc., 1972.

SCHACTER, D. L. The hypnagogic state: a critical review of the literature. *Psychological Bulletin,* 1976, 83, 3: 452-481.

SCHAFER, R. *Aspects of internalization.* New York: International Universities Press, 1968.

SCHNECK, J. M. Personality components in patients with sleep paralysis. *Psychiatric Quarterly,* 1969, 43: 343-348.

SLIGHT, D. Hypnagogic phenomena. *Journal of Abnormal Psychology,* 1924, 19: 274-282.

SMITH, C. Psychosomatic aspects of narcolepsy. *Journal of Mental Science,* 1958, 104: 593-607.

SOURS, J. Narcolepsy and other disturbances in the sleep waking rhythm: a study of 115 cases with review of the literature. *Journal of Nervous and Mental Disease,* 1963, 137: 525-542.

STROEBEL, C. F. The importance of biological clocks in mental health. *Mental Health Progress Reports-2.* Public Health Service Publication #1743. Chevy Chase, Md.: National Institute of Mental Health, 1968, 323-351.

SZATMARI, A. and HACHE, I. Narcolepsy: clinical, electrophysiological and biochemical appraisal. *Electroencephalography and Clinical Neurophysiology,* 1962, 14: 586-587.

TAKAHASHI, S. The action of Tricyclics (alone or in combination with Methylphemidate) upon several symptoms of narcolepsy. In: Guilleminault, C., Dement, W. C., and Passouant, P. (Eds.), *Narcolepsy: Advances in sleep research, Vol. 3.* New York: Spectrum Publications, 1976.

THARP, R. Narcolepsy and epilepsy. In: Guilleminault, C., Dement, W. C., and Passouant, P. (Eds.), *Narcolepsy: Advances in sleep research, Vol. 3.* New York: Spectrum Publications, 1976.

THAYER, R. E. Measurement of activation through self-report. *Psychological Reports,* 1967, 20: 663-678.

VAN TWYVER, H. B. Sleep patterns of five rodent species. *Physiological Behavior,* 1969, 4: 901-905.

VIHVELIN, H. On the differentiation of some typical forms of hypnagogic hallucinations. *Acta Psychiatrica et Neurologica,* 1948, 23: 359-389.

VOGEL, G. W. Studies in the psychophysiology of dreams: III. The dream of narcolepsy. *Archives of General Psychiatry,* 1960, 3: 421-425.

VOGEL, G. W. et al. REM sleep reduction effects on depression syndromes. *Archives of General Psychiatry,* 1975, 32: 765-777.

WARE, J. C. The symptom of insomnia: causes and cures. *Psychiatric Annals,* 1979, 9, 7: 27-49.

WEBB, W. B. Individual differences in sleep length. In: Hartmann, E. (Ed.), *Sleep and dreaming.* Boston: Little Brown and Co., 1970.

WEBB, W. B. and AGNEW, H. W., JR. Measurement and characteristics of nocturnal sleep. In: Abt, L. A. and Riess, B. F., (Eds.), *Progress in clinical psychology,* Vol. 8, New York: Grune & Stratton, 1969.

WEITZMAN, E. D. Twenty-four hour neuroendocrine secretory patterns: observations on patients with narcolepsy. In: Guilleminault, C., Dement, W. C., and Passouant, P. (Eds.), *Narcolepsy: Advances in sleep research, Vol. 3.* New York: Spectrum Publications, 1976.

WEITZMAN, E. D., BOYAR, R. M., KAPEN, S. and HELLMAN, L. The relationship of sleep and sleep stages to neuroendocrine secretion and biological rhythms in man. *Recent Progress in Hormone Research,* 1975, 31: 399-446.

WEITZNER, H. A. Sleep paralysis successfully treated with insulin hypoglycemia. *Archives of Neurology and Psychiatry,* 1952, 68: 835.

WILLIAMS, R. L. and KARACAN, I. Clinical disorders of sleep. In: Usdin, G. (Ed.), *Sleep research and clinical practice.* New York: Brunner/Mazel, 1973.

WILLIAMS, R. L., KARACAN, I., and HIRSCH, C. *Electroencephalography (EEG) of human sleep: Clinical applications.* New York: John Wiley & Sons, 1974.

WILLIAMS, R. L., WARE, J. C., ILANIA, R. L. and KARACAN, I. Disturbed sleep and anxiety. In: Fann, W. E., et al. (Eds.) *Phenomenology and treatment of anxiety.* New York: Spectrum Publications, 1979.

WINNICOTT, D. W. Transitional objects and transitional phenomena. *International Journal of Psychoanalysis,* 1953, 34: 89-97.

WINNICOTT, D. W. *Collected papers.* New York: Basic Books; London: Tavistock, 1958.

WOLBERG, L. R. *Medical hypnosis.* Vol. I and II. New York: Grune & Stratton, 1948.

WRETMARK, G. A study in grief reactions. *Acta Psychiatrica et Neurologica Scandinavia,* 1959, 136.

YOSS, R. E. and DALY, D. D. Criteria for the diagnosis of the narcoleptic syndrome. *Proceedings of Staff Meetings, Mayo Clinic,* 1957, 32:320-328.

YOSS, R. E. and DALY, D. D. Treatment of narcolepsy with Ritalin. *Neurology,* 1959, 9: 171.

YOSS R. E. and DALY, D. D. Hereditary aspects of narcolepsy. *Transamerican Neurological Association,* 1960, 85: 239-240.

ZARCONE, V. Narcolepsy. *New England Journal of Medicine,* 1973, 228: 1156-1166.

ZARCONE, V. P. Sleep and schizophrenia. *Psychiatric Annals,* August, 1979, 8, 9: 385-402.

ZUNG, W. W. K. The treatment of insomnia with anti-depressant drugs. *Psychophysiology,* 1968, 5: 234.

ZUNG, W. W. K. The pharmacology of disordered sleep. In: Hartmann, E. (Ed.), *Sleep and dreaming.* Boston: Little Brown and Co., 1970.

ZUNG, W. W. K. and WILSON, W. P. Sleep and dream patterns in twins. In: Wortis, J. (Ed.), *Recent advances in biological psychiatry.* Vol. 9, New York: Plenum Press, 1967.

ZUNG, W. W. K., WILSON, W. P. and DODSON, W. E. Effect of depressive disorders on sleep EEG responses. *Archives of General Psychiatry,* 1964, 10: 439-445.

Index